2

AF528640

American HIV/AIDS Narratives
Disease and the Question of Identity

American HIV/AIDS Narratives

Disease and the Question of Identity

Maniklal Bhanja

ADHYAYAN

ADHYAYAN PUBLISHERS&DISTRIBUTORS
New Delhi-110002

Published by
ADHYAYAN PUBLISHERS & DISTRIBUTORS
4378/4B, 105, J.M.D. House, Murari Lal Street
Ansari Road Darya Ganj, New Delhi - 110002
Ph.: 011-23263018, 011-23277156, Fax: 23280028
Email: adhyayanpublishers@yahoo.com

American HIV/AIDS Narratives
Disease and the Question of Identity

© Author
Edition 2011
ISBN 978-81-8435-299-3

The responsibility for facts stated, opinion expressed or conclusions reached and plagiarism, if any, in this book is entirely that of the author/editor. The publisher bears no responsibility for them whatsoever.

Printed in India

Published by Harish Chandra Yadav for Adhyayan Publishers & Distributors, Delhi. Laser Typesetting at Jain Computers and Printed at Tarun Offset Printers, Delhi

To

Professor Dilip Kumar Das,

my teacher and mentor

Preface

Even though disease is scientifically understood to have been communicated mainly through bacteria or viruses, infections, contagions and transmission routes, it is also passed through malady-based discourses and practices that in effect construct illness. While investigating the 1832 cholera epidemic in Paris, Francois Delaporte, a French researcher, in his book *Disease and Civilization: The Cholera in Paris, 1832* (trans. Arthur Goldhammer, Cambridge, MIT Press, 1986.) writes, "I assert, to begin with, that 'disease' does not exist. It is therefore illusory to think that one can 'develop beliefs' about it to 'respond' to it. What does exist is not disease but practices" (6). Delaporte's statement, of course, does not derecognize actuality of disease, suffering and death. Rather, it draws attention to construction of illness through multiple representations, responses and conceptualizations. It focuses on the cultural production of disease and on the people's consumption of myths surrounding sickness. It also suggests that how rational response to disease is always ignored. Thus, it tries to highlight what might be called disease-centric cultural criticism.

In the light of the implications of Delaporte's assertion, I have framed the central argument of this book. I have argued that even as disease is experienced in the body individually, it is simultaneously cultural in its effects, since its implication is understood and represented by the community, nation and world in terms of medical, ethical and political issues that consequently address the question of identity of the diseased. This key argument has been developed by studying different cultural perceptions and interpretations of diseases in general and the HIV/AIDS epidemic in particular. It has been made stronger by taking a close look at some of the American HIV/AIDS Narratives of the 1980s and 1990s.

HIV/AIDS is a disease that requires both clinical and nonclinical interventions to curb its spread. In this book, I seek to intervene nonmedically and intellectually as well in the popular perception of the disease as stigma. By adopting interdisciplinary approach to the subject of disease, I have tried to show that HIV/AIDS entails more an epistemological question than a moral one. I have critiqued different cultural notions and practices concerning the AIDS epidemic, and have demonstrated that our tendency to label and stigmatize HIV positive people issues out of our ideologies and prejudices that are often normative or regulatory or political rather than rational or nonjudgmental or apolitical.

In Chapter-I an attempt has been made to see disease, identity and narrative in relation to the HIV/AIDS epidemic. Cultural representations concerning disease and HIV/AIDS, which have been studied from sociological perspectives by different critics have been paid attention to. The notion of identity has then been viewed from linguistic and psychoanalytic angles. A compromise between essentialism and constructionism has been arrived at to understand the gendered, sexualised and diseased bodies that suffer. This has been linked up with identity-related questions that HIV/AIDS raises. The fact that identity is mediated through narrative has been discussed. Chapter-I, by and large, seeks to provide a sort of *cultural theory of disease and HIV-positive identity.* Chapter-II discusses the question of HIV-positive identity in American HIV/AIDS nonfiction that includes history, biography and autobiography. Chapter-III attempts to examine HIV-positive identity in hegemonic American HIV/AIDS fiction. Chapter-IV seeks to look at HIV-positive identity in counter-hegemonic American HIV/AIDS fiction. Chapter-V tries to summarize the preceding chapters and concludes with an ethical note that this book primarily aims at. Certainly this book will not help cure patients, let alone HIV-positive people. However, I trust, it will help people understand the diseased with love and care. Where there is the body, there is illness. We are frail and likely to suffer from diseases, yet we love to engage in pointing the accusing finger at the diseased.

I am grateful to the library staff of the Indo-American Centre for International Studies (formerly American Studies Research Center), Hyderabad and of the Indian Institute of Technology (IIT) Central Library, Guwahati for assisting me in getting some of the materials pertaining to this project photocopied. My participation in the Theory/Praxis course organized by the Forum on Contemporary Theory, Baroda in 2005 at IIT Guwahati helped me develop new insights into my study. I would like to thank my teacher, Dr. Prafulla C Kar, Director, Centre for Contemporary Theory, Vadodara and Former Professor of English, The Maharaja Sayajirao University of Baroda for allowing me to participate in the course.

My acknowledgment must certainly go to Dr. Rajagopalan Radhakrishnan, Professor of English and Comparative Literature at the University of California-Irvine for his suggestions. I owe my debt of thanks to Gloria Miklowitz, Penny Raife Durant and Charlotte Watson Sherman for the gift copies of their novels concerning HIV/AIDS. I am indebted to my friend, Professor Gregg de Young of the American University in Cairo for sending me some xeroxed materials.

I am grateful to J N Choudhury (the former principal), Dr. Charu Saharia Nath (the present principal), my former colleagues (especially Dr. Suresh K Arya and Dr. Abdul

Mazid) of Tezpur College (Assam), Professor Ranjit Kumar Dev Goswami of Gauhati University, Dr K N Prabhu of IITGuwahati, Dr Dilip Naik of English and Foreign Languages University, Hyderabad, Dr Nigamananda Das of Nagaland University, and Dr Nalini Kanta Samanta, of Ganjam Law College, Berhampur (Orissa) for their rock-like support to traverse unhindered the trajectories of my engagement in writing the book.

Thanks are also due to Hareswar Nath, Dilip Burman, Mala Burman, Murchhana Bhattacharjee, Akani Barua (Mami), Naresh Thakur, Puran Chandra Kalita, Khanindra Mazumdar, Dr. Jyotsna Sharma Bezbarua, Dr. Dwipen Mahanta, Raju Pokhrel, Saroj Kumar Samanta and Ramanath Das who have always non-judgmentally and unconditionally come forward with their big-hearted gestures for the management of my crises faced during the period of my writing this book. To thank my awe-inspiring friend, Ankur Acharya, assistant editor with the publication division of Sangeet Natak Akademi (New Delhi) for his consistently sincere love and care to promote my intellectual pursuits will be an understatement. I want to thank my wife, Sarita for her utmost care during the long writing process.

I am grateful to Natwar Thakkar, editor of *Ishani* and Dr. Jacob Kani, editor of *Indian Currents* for publishing my articles concerning HIV/AIDS that, after revisions, have been incorporated in the present book. I would like to extend my deep gratitude to Harish Chandra Yadav of Adhyayan publishers (New Delhi) for bringing my manuscript into its present shape.

Tezpur
March, 2011

Maniklal Bhanja

Contents

1

Seeing Disease, Identity and Narrative in Relation to HIV/AIDS

Focussing on HIV/AIDS, this chapter attempts to examine the notion of disease and identity. It also seeks to look at the representation and politics of the illness. It argues for the importance and necessity of narratives to cope with the questions of HIV-positive identity.

I

The term "disease" is defined as an unhealthy condition of the body or the mind. Usually the absence of "disease" is understood to constitute "health" - "health" that is foreknown, predetermined to be whole, hence privileged and desirable, which is why, as John Donne in his prose work *Devotions Upon Emergent Occasions* puts it, "We study Health, and we deliberate upon our meats, and drink, and ayre, and exercises, [...] and so our Health is a long and a regular work" (417). According to the Austrian-born English philosopher Ludwig Wittgenstein (who died of cancer), even though painful bodily processes involved both in healthiness and unhealthiness are almost identical, "no one wants to put a disease on the same level as normal life [and no one wants to speak of disease as if it had the same rights as healthy bodily processes (even painful ones)]" (20e). He argues further that it is possible to regard disease in the body as "natural" if the whole feeling of the people and the nation for the body changes. Wittgenstein's argument points to the fact that health is always already out there as the dominant and hegemonic concept. This is how health is culturally mapped out.

In this preconceived wholeness of health, disease is a split and is known in and through its social and cultural practices that are predominantly medical, ethical and political. The medical is connected with the practice of diagnosis, treatment and prevention of disease. Thus, the clinical aspects of illness involve technological discovery of microorganisms, antibodies, pathological signs or symptoms, infections, routes of transmission, treatment of illness and epidemiology. The ethical is concerned with goodness or badness and accepted rules of human character or behaviour, and with the distinction between right and wrong. The moral aspects of sickness involve stigmatization, status degradation, identity transformation (the disabled body) and labelling or categorizing. The political relates to the state, government or public affairs, to the ideas, policies or strategies of and the competition between the different parties or groups engaging in the activities involved both in getting or using power in public life and in being able to influence decisions that affect a country or society. It is also connected with something that is done, with disregard of principle, in the interests of status, power, etc. within an organization or group, and with something that is motivated by a person's beliefs or actions concerning politics. Thus, the political refers to an activity or space that is objectified through a position or status, a person or group and an institution or organization. The political features of illness include the practices of discrimination, marginalization of disease and the exercise of power over them, and also, the engagement in countercharges and counteractions to pursue ideology-based and self-interested aims. The politics of disease is manifested through accusation and activism (resistance).

These practices that will be examined in their interrelatedness later in this chapter are the established ways in which societies respond to disease and consequently conceptualize, represent and interpret the state of being unwell in body or mind. In so doing, they define only the lack of that preformulated wholeness of health. Out of these practices, the "clinical" is the preferred choice and is accepted as the general perception of disease in modern times. However, its supreme scientific status over the humanistic in disease discourse has been questioned following the AIDS epidemic.

Acquired Immune Deficiency Syndrome (AIDS) is caused by a retrovirus called the human immunodeficiency virus (HIV) of "unknown" origin. HIV is transmitted through body fluids (blood, sexual fluids and breast milk), leading to a severe loss of immunity and leaving the sufferer susceptible to infection. Explaining what HIV does in the body, the World Health Organization (WHO) notes, "our body has white blood cells which fight against disease germs and kill them. Thus, white blood cells protect us from falling sick. When a person has HIV in the body, the virus destroys the white blood cells which then can no longer fight against disease germs. This makes the person sick"(3). These white blood cells are called Thymus lymphocytes or T-cells. Immediately after its transmission in the bloodstream, HIV incorporates itself within the genetic structure of a specific T-cell that is not killed but rendered non-functional. Remaining dormant, it then gradually uses the material of the cell to manufacture millions of copies of itself before the cell's death. These newly created HIVs locate other healthy T-cells in the bloodstream to resume their process of replication and destruction. The virus is extremely labile and has a ten-year-plus incubation period. Dryness, simplest sterilization and the mildest disinfectants can destroy HIV outside the body system.

HIV impairs the immune system and thereby causes opportunities for other infections or diseases. The term AIDS refers to a complex of disease conditions like fever, rash, diarrhoea, weight loss, lymphadenopathy (swelling of lymph nodes), a rare skin cancer called Kaposi's Sarcoma, a form of pneumonia called Pneumocystis Carinii Pneumonia (PCP), candidiasis (yeast infection), cryptococcus meningitis and tuberculosis. Symptoms vary from one location to another, from country to country. People affected by HIV/AIDS are also susceptible to the infections/diseases that are already present in any given geography. One gradually succumbs to the virus and the syndrome manifested in a nexus of diseases. People with intact immune system are not normally affected by HIV/AIDS-related diseases. Thus, HIV/AIDS in itself is transmissible but not contagious. It is a condition of an ever-changing group of concurrent pathological signs or symptoms. At the moment there is no accurate treatment, no known cure for the disease, even though scientific communities the world over are engaged in developing a vaccine.

As of now, routes of transmission of HIV/AIDS are believed to be sexual (anal or vaginal) intercourse, blood transfusion, use of infected injection or surgical equipment such as needles, blades or razors and from infected mother to child. There is also some risk of transmission through breast milk. As soon as HIV enters the human body, the individual becomes infectious, that is, he or she can infect other people with HIV. The symptomatological nature and eventual fatalness of HIV/AIDS have been a cause for major concern in the medical community.

What is now known as HIV/AIDS was first recognized as a disease among "white" homosexual males in USA in 1981. As early as 1979, doctors in New York, Los Angeles and San Francisco had observed their young gay male patients with long term swelling of lymph nodes, pneumocystis carinii pneumonia (PCP) and Kaposi's Sarcoma (KS), which were similar to those seen among Central Africans and elderly men of Mediterranean origin. These diseases were linked to immune deficiency, and the complex was initially designated AID (Acquired Immune Deficiency), ACIDS (Acquired Community Immune Deficiency Syndrome) or GRID (Gay-Related Immune Deficiency). After the identification of more symptoms, diseases and germs in non-gays like intravenous drug users, haemophiliacs and Haitians, the Centers for Disease Control (CDC) in Atlanta adopted the neutral acronym AIDS (Acquired Immune Deficiency Syndrome) in 1982. Only at a later stage was it recognized that heterosexuals were also susceptible to the disease. The virus that caused AIDS was initially named LAV (lymphadenopathy-associated virus) by Luc Montagnier of the Pasteur Institute, France in 1983. It was subsequently named HTLV-III (human T-cell lymphotropic virus type III) by Robert Gallo of the National Cancer Institute, USA in 1984. It was once again named ARV (AIDS-associated retrovirus) by Dr. Jay Levy of the University of California, San Francisco, USA in 1984. The Centers for Disease Control (CDC) adopted the joint name LAV/HTLV-III and HTLV-III/LAV as a peacekeeping formula for scientific communities in France and USA. It was popularly known as the AIDS virus by the press, and finally named HIV (human immunodeficiency virus) as a unifying formula in May 1986. The World Health Organization (WHO) recommends the acronym HIV/AIDS to rise above all disputes pertaining to the naming of the virus and the disease. It may also be mentioned here that Luc Montagnier and Francoise Barre-Sinoussi, two French scientists won half the 2008 Nobel Prize for medicine or physiology (the other half of the prize was shared by Harald zur Hausen, a German cancer researcher) for discovering and identifying the deadly virus.

This brief account of HIV/AIDS shows the succession of discursive naming and categories, a succession that has been informed by the medical model of the disease in one register. In the other register, transmissibility of the disease through "unsafe" heterosexual or homosexual sex has most significantly problematized desire and pleasure as well as the body and the mind of the human being, since it is impossible to give up sex. This latter position is perhaps the single most important reason as to why HIV/AIDS, with its ineluctable association with stigma and death has drastically changed the ways of seeing disease in recent years and thereby occasions an ever-shifting semantic crisis over disease in general. The canonical privilege of biomedicine in regard to the "meaning" of disease is critiqued in humanities and social sciences. As Thomas E. Yingling in an unpaginated article in *AIDS and the National Body* puts it, "it is the question of reading with uncertain terms that AIDS forces upon us."

The justification for such multidisciplinary approaches to disease lies perhaps in the notion of what W.J.T. Mitchell calls, "a hard, rigorous relativism that regards knowledge as a social product, a matter of dialogue between different versions of the world, including different languages, ideologies, and modes of representation" (*Iconology* 38). Relativism is the doctrine that holds that knowledge is relative, not absolute or objective and universally valid. It considers any knowledge as having significance in relation to something else, as implying comparison or contextual relationship, as involving a different but corresponding idea. In other words, relativism is a difference in similarity between things or terms in the world of knowledge produced by society. Thus, the knowledge of a thing or a person is understood in terms of another and eternally tends to be indeterminate. That is why all types of episteme, be it personal, esoteric or exoteric, need to be approached holistically for appropriate understanding.

Hence, the knowledge of disease following the HIV/AIDS epidemic has been seen as something that is individual and sociocultural at the same time. Like the interpretive convention of any community or nation, the present experience of disease is looked at in the light of its significant (mostly catastrophic) pastness or historicity coupled with the self-conscious theoretical practices of knowledge of sickness by the medical profession and society as well. These methodological symbolic readings of pathological signs are represented as something having similiarity to the original symptoms, and work to provide eventually, to quote Sander L. Gilman, "the set of associations, which [...] doctors, patients, or observers subconsciously apply to the idea of specific diseases" (7). In this process disease is assigned a name that is validated officially and, in due course, communally.

II

HIV/AIDS has caused, as Yingling argues, an "asymptotic space," "a gap between the apprehension and the comprehension of the disease [...]" (38). This state of the disease, as has been shown above in the brief account of HIV/AIDS, is always supplemented or substituted with something, creates difference and deferral in the epistemic status of its "meaning" objectified and communicated in "representation."

Representation is defined as the act of standing for or corresponding to something or someone that once again stands for or acts for a whole group of things or persons by consensual agreement. In fact the notion of representation, be it semiotic or political, is always elastic, open-ended and essentially symbolic. In semiotic theories of representation, the representational material (object or form) is called the "signifier," while the concept (idea or referent) which that material evokes is designated as the "signified." In order to represent something, human beings establish relationships between the signifier and the signified in iconic, indexical and symbolic ways. The iconic shows resemblance. The indexical stresses cause-and-effect relationship (for example, visual things like cinematic and photographic images are both iconic and indexical.). The symbolic stipulates arbitrariness without having any resemblance. In this process, as against the Swiss linguist Ferdinand de Saussure's linguistic norm that "sign" arbitrarily unites a sound-image (signifier, for instance "tree") and a concept (signified, e.g. the sound-image/word "tree" conjures up in people's minds the idea or picture of "tree."), the commutability of the signified is continuously attained. As the French philosopher Jacques Derrida cogently argues, "[...] the signified always already functions as a signifier [...]. There is not a single signified that escapes [...] the play of signifying references that constitute language" (7). In many ways, as Kaja Silverman has shown, "one signified always gives way to another, functions in its turn as a signifier" (38). This is precisely the process of signification. In political form of representation where persons act for other persons, there is also a flexible interaction between the citizens and the government. Thus, in both forms of representation is inherent a shifting or unstable relationship to authentic "meaning" of knowledge or experience that is endlessly constituted by what it is not. Talking about "experience" Jonathan Culler says, "[...] it has always already occurred and yet is still to be produced - an indispensable point of reference, yet never simply there" (63).

Thus, every representation is a misrecognition of the "original or authentic." W.J.T.Mitchell in his essay "Representation" appropriately remarks, "Representation is that by which we make our will known and, simultaneously, that which alienates our will from ourselves [...]. Every representation exacts some cost, in the form of lost immediacy, presence, or truth, in the form of a gap between intention and realization, original and copy [...]. Sometimes it is as ample as the gap between life and death" (21). This "gap" consequently creates an "illusion" of a thing *per se* in the representational world. These endless illusions that influence and are influenced by stimuli emerging from within and without the individual are constantly constructed and organized as schemata that possibly seek to serve as, to quote Joseph Sandler, "the background frame of reference to all current processes of perception, imagining, remembering, feeling, and thinking"(qtd. in Gilman 1). These schemata are once again subject to revisionism in the course of human experience. In other words, as the American philosopher Charles Sanders Peirce argues, "The meaning of a representation can be nothing but a representation" (1:171).

In this scheme of perpetually open-ended representation mediated through language, everything including disease always acquires meanings or significations. HIV/AIDS has also continually been proliferating viral, personal, communal, national and global histories and allegories in its semiotic and political forms of representations. Through the mass media, as Cindy Patton puts it, "the virus itself becomes a character - the little hunk of protein that refuses to give up its secrets. 'Perhaps the virus is trying to tell us something,' both new right doomsday prophets and scientists have said" (*Inventing* 25-6). Referring to the battles over the continual change in the meanings and names of the virus, a change that has accompanied every stage of research and treatment, Paula A. Triechler calls HIV/AIDS an epidemic of a transmissible lethal disease and an epidemic of meanings or significations. She uses the term "epidemic" to refer to the exponential compounding of meanings as opposed to the simpler spread of a term through population and applies the term "signification" in the linguistic sense. She writes, "Many scientists and physicians, even those sensitive to the complexities of AIDS, believe that 'the fact' ('science' or 'reason') will resolve contradiction and supplant speculation; they express impatience with social interpretations, which they perceive as superfluous or incorrect [...]. Signification processes are not the handmaidens of 'the facts', rather 'the facts' themselves arise out of the signifying practices of biomedical discourse" (331). In a similar fashion, Thomas Yingling writes, "AIDS [...] can be apprehended - on bodies, in friends, in news reports, in changing populations, behaviors, and rituals: we know that it is in some undeniable sense 'real,' whether its reality be outside or within us. But the frames of intelligibility that provide it with even a meager measure of comprehensibility are notoriously unstable. [...] the quotidian meaning of AIDS seems to change almost as often as the virus itself replicates [...]" (38). In its potential for decentring its centre or origin, HIV/AIDS has most justifiably been called a postmodern disease in the Derridean sense. In fact, as Karen Atkinson and Rob Middlehurst in their essay "Representing AIDS: the textual politics of health discourse" put it, "AIDS constitutes a site for a discursive struggle for meanings" (115).

This engenders tensions between the material reality (a tiny virus) and the linguistic portrayal (shifts in sociocultural perception) and, as a result, spawns mythopoeic discourses about HIV/AIDS. For example, the tsunami in the Indian Ocean on December 26, 2004, which killed nearly two lakh people, had been compared to the "devastation wreaked by the virus all over the world" (8). The *Times of India,* a daily newspaper in its January 8, 2005 edition had put the headline of its editorial thus: "Viral Tsunami: Unchecked HIV epidemic could destroy countries." The editorial related to the death of a niece, two grand-nephews and son of South African President Nelson Mandela from HIV/AIDS that was also, at that point of time, killing at least one thousand people every day. African archbishop Desmond Tutu said that it was an affliction more devastating than apartheid.

Discussing the tropes of disease discourse in the West, Susan Sontag in her book *AIDS and Its Metaphors* refers to military metaphors like "invasion," "invaders," "enemy," "battlefield" and "war" respectively for disease, microorganisms, the ill, the body and efforts to minimize mortality rate from disease. Sontag analyses leprosy, syphilis, cholera, cancer and plague as metaphorized illnesses that give those affected by them new identities through the transformation of their bodies and faces into something alienating. The manifestation of these illnesses and sexually transmitted diseases (STDs) like syphilis in particular in different periods of the history of disease is described and hence perceived by doctors, religious leaders and bureaucrats as "collective calamity, evil, scourge," "the wrath of God," "punishment," "pollution" and "plague." Added to these metaphors that also flourish around HIV/AIDS are ascriptions like "the revenge of nature," "the gay plague," "corruption," "catastrophe" and "apocalypse." The HIV/AIDS condition has been referred to as something that is "terrifying," "stigmatizing," "dehumanizing," "disempowering" and "disgusting." The risk-groups are treated as "the exotic, primitive," "others," "the foreign," "the non-us, the alien" and "a community of pariahs" (Sontag 45-87). This metaphoric factor with its militaristic connotation entrenches the notion of disease as invasion. According to Sontag, "The metaphorized illnesses that haunt the collective imagination are all hard deaths, or envisaged as such. Being deadly is not in itself enough to produce terror" (38). Sontag argues that the effect of the military imagery is far-reaching: "It overmobilizes, it overdescribes, and it powerfully contributes to the excommunicating and stigmatizing of the ill" (94). In exposing, criticizing, belaboring and using up military metaphors she seeks liberation from the constraints of the martial ethos of HIV/AIDS tropes. She finds this ethically consoling. For her, "the medical model of the public weal [...] not only provides a persuasive justification for authoritarian rule but implicitly suggests the necessity of state-sponsored repression and violence [...]" (94).

The different names of the virus such as LAV, HTLV-III, ARV, LAV/HTLV-III or HTLV-III/LAV, AIDS virus and HIV are another instance of signification. The epidemiological model that categorized high-risk groups (rather than high-risk practices) such as the "4-H list" (homosexuals, haemophiliacs, heroin addicts and Haitians) and "prostitutes," rather than "heterosexuals" who were initially excluded as forming a category susceptible also to HIV/AIDS, is yet another instance. This is the reason why Steven F. Kruger argues, "Diseases often, perhaps always, take on social and cultural meanings that make it possible for them to be seen not just as random events, but as part of some plan or meaningful pattern [...]. Molecular biology, in its most basic terms and concepts, metaphorizes its subject matter as language" (23). Such shifts in signification in the dominant scientistic or medical "language" and "intention" also influence, even shape the perception of HIV/AIDS at all levels. As Cindy Patton in *Globalizing AIDS* has put it, "The methodical nature of Western medicine and the degree to which modern society is medicalized means that without the procedures and sanctions of official medicine, expressions of bodily experiences and complaints are not considered real, sometimes not even by the sufferer"(xxiii). Thus, the constant circulation of these terms in hegemonic discourse constructs stereotypes of disease and the diseased, stereotypes that in turn serve as the fixed models for imagining sickness and for labelling the sufferers of sickness. The above argument on HIV/AIDS discourse highlights the "language" of representation and shows, as the French philosopher Paul Ricouer would maintain, "Language, indeed, is constituted in such a way that it does not condemn us to the choice [...] between the conceptual or the ineffable"(27).

III

The representational dynamics of disease discourse must be understood in terms of human identity, since it is in and through representation that identities, including diseased ones, are constituted. Human beings, unlike other animals, are instinctively representational. It is within representation that people imagine, visualize and recognize themselves and thereby produce identities. Talking about the key role that representation plays in human life, Kath Woodword says, "This is how we signal our identities to others and how we know which people we identify with and those who are distinguished as being different" (12). Moreover, HIV/AIDS discourse has highlighted the overarching question of identity in a most articulate manner, since it focuses on a palpable/ objective live "body" conducting itself promiscuously through unfulfillable desire and pleasure to death. Simon Watney in *Policing Desire: Pornography, AIDS, and the Media* writes, "AIDS is not only a medical crisis on an unparalleled scale, it involves a crisis of representation itself, a crisis over the entire framing of knowledge about the human body and its capacities for sexual pleasure" (9). This is why it is crucial to address the problematics of identity (,problematics in which is also most prominently implicated "the body" that has been gendered, sexualized and politicized) in relation to HIV/ AIDS. However, first of all, it is imperative to understand "identity."

"Identity" as a term is derived from the Latin word *idem* meaning the "same." It is defined in two ways: the first refers to the quality or condition of being a specified person or thing, to individuality, personality; and the second relates to identification, to the state of being identical, of being the same in substance, nature, qualities, etc. The first definition focuses on the innate, unified and fixed notion of identity. It is essentialist in the sense that it is founded on, as Diana Fuss shows, "a belief in true essence - that which is most irreducible, unchanging, and therefore constitutive of a given person or thing" (2). In this view, identity is inborn, naturally given, pure, uncoded and cannot be constructed or reconstructed - that is to say, one is born with an identity.

The second definition points to the interactive and constructed notion of "identification" as an act of associating oneself with another or of regarding oneself as sharing characteristics of another. It entails active engagement with a position by the one who takes up identities. One has to consciously or unconsciously identify with, has to be recruited into an identity position. As Paul Ricoeur argues, "To identify something is to be able to make apparent to others, amid a range of particular things of the same type, of *which* one we intend to speak" (27). One has to perform an identity. It is constructionist in the sense that "the natural is itself posited as a construction of the social" (Fuss 3). However, sociality always changes and in the process differences are produced and organized. This leads to the question of interrelationship between social "structures" (dynamics beyond human control which shape and exercise constraint over identities) and individual "agency" (degree of intervention and control one can exert over one's participation or choice in construction of identities). Identity is thus constituted by the interaction between the public or social meanings on the one hand and personal experience (subjective evaluations and choices) on the other. To identify with a group or nation by sharing is called collective identity. Identity is a configuration of differences and similarities across collectivities or individuals. Simply put, "Identity is marked by similarity, that is of the people like us, and by difference, of those who are not" (Woodward 7). It is defined by what one is not, by the other, by the difference that relationally involves oppositions or inequalities. From this viewpoint, identity is always in the process of being made or formed and can be reconstructed.

The problem of identity, as Avrum Stroll sees it, "may be thought of as the problem of trying to give a true explanation of those features of the world which account for its sameness, on the one hand, and for its diversity and change, on the other [...]. Difficulties about identity lie at the heart of a vast corpus of seemingly unrelated problems" (121). Difficulties about "identity" at the conceptual level need to be looked at somewhat deeply in consideration of the issues that HIV/AIDS discourse raises in this connection.

"Identity" of the individual was first described in the 17th century French philosopher Rene Descartes's dictum "I think, therefore I am" (well known in its Latin formulation, *"Cogito, ergo sum,"* though originally written in French, "Je pense, donc je suis"). "I" is the self or the human subject. Thinking establishes existence of a person. Mind (thinking)-body (matter) dualism expressed as mind controlling body is precisely the Cartesian model of human identity. Identity of the Cartesian human subject established by the fact of its thinking or awareness was centred on individual "consciousness" that was considered to be the origin of knowledge, meaning and action. Contrary to this belief, the post-Cartesian existence of a being is predominantly shaped by "language" and by psychoanalysis with its stress on "the unconscious."

The human subject uses "language" and is defined by means of it. Language manifests itself through "signs" expressing ideas or meanings. Along with the semiotic model of Ferdinand de Saussure, the semiotic scheme of Charles Sanders Peirce describes the human subject as the product of language, as cognitively experiencing the world through language. He writes, "[...] the word or sign which man uses *is* the man himself. [...] the fact that every thought is a sign, taken in conjunction with the fact that life is a train of thought, proves that man is a sign. [...] the man and the [...] sign are identical [...]. Thus my language is the sum total of myself; for the man is the thought" (5: 189). Man and his thought as well are at once a sign and a signifier. By linking closely language and human consciousness, Peirce here insists that people's sense of themselves and of the world outside is only accessed by semiotic process. Peirce's model is open-ended in its treatment of signs, and by extension, of identity and is, therefore, against the Saussurean one.

The logocentricity of the Saussurean model seeks to define the linguistic "sign" as the "arbitrary" (not natural) combination of the signifier (form) and the signified (concept that form evokes), both being without any identity outside the linguistic convention. Sign possesses meaning by virtue of it being different from any other sign without any linguistic reason. The word "house" is the signifier and the concept of "house" is the signified. Between them there is no natural link outside the linguistic system to explain the meaning of house. A word is identified only through its relationship with and difference from other words in the system of language. Meaning emanates from linguistic "differences" without any positive terms. Saussure's model operates within a closed domain of signification. It, however, suggests that language speaks individuals, rather than individuals speak language. Language situates people in different social contexts and thereby constructs their identities. People know themselves within language. Saussure indirectly makes a case for somewhat fixed construction of identity. This Structuralist notion of structuring of human identity in and through language has been taken up by Emile Benveniste who, insisting on the subjective foundations of language argues:

> It is in and through language that man constitutes himself as a *subject*, because language alone establishes the concept of "ego" in reality, in *its* reality which is that of the being.
>
> The "subjectivity" [...] is the capacity of the speaker to posit himself as "subject." It is defined not by the feeling which everyone experiences of being himself [...] but as the psychic unity that transcends the totality of the actual experiences it assembles and that makes the permanence of

> the consciousness. Now we hold that that "subjectivity," [...] is only the emergence in the being of a fundamental property of language. "Ego" is he who *says* "ego." That is where we see the foundation of "subjectivity," which is determined by the linguistic status of "person." (224)

Benveniste treats language (langue), discourse (parole) and subjectivity (a grammatical entity and a speaker) "inseparably." He believes that the cultural identity of the individual is possible only within discourse, only by means of the pronouns "I" and "you" that are for him, signifiers without conventional signifieds. Person identifies with the first and is defined in opposition to the second. As Kaja Silverman notes, "the signifier 'I' always implies a speaker, to whom it refers. Similarly, the signifier 'you' always implies a listener, to whom the speaker talks. These roles are endlessly reversible, as are the signifiers which depend upon them; the person who functions as a speaker for one moment functions as a listener for the next. They are also only intermittently activated, as a consequence of which the signifiers 'I' and 'you' have only a periodic meaning" (44). In this discursive process these pronouns subsequently lose their significance. The speaking subject is the agency of discourse. The subject of speech is the discursive element. The spoken subject is the subject produced through discourse. For Benveniste, the subject remains indistinguishable from signification and is provisional by being continuously reconstructed through discourse such as conversation, film, the mass media, internet, photography and so on. In discourse between two persons, one addresses the other and in the process defines oneself and hence gains "identity." Benveniste's linguistic model is closely linked to the interpellation model of the French Marxist philosopher Louis Althusser.

In Althusser, discourse takes place between an

individual and a socioculturally constructed (even determined) identity position or agent that is ideological. The latter addresses the former and defines in the process much of the former's identity. This address is what Althusser calls "hailing" or "interpellation" that is described as an operation or process whereby people are consciously or unconsciously compelled to recognize themselves in a particular identity through identifying themselves with the representations that their culture provides. In his essay "Ideology and Ideological State Apparatuses," he writes, "ideology 'acts' or 'functions' in such a way that it 'recruits' subjects among the individuals (it recruits them all) or 'transforms' the individuals into subjects (it transforms them all) by [...] *interpellation* or hailing [...]" (130). When the policeman, for instance, hails "Hey, you there!", the hailed individual will turn round thinking "yes, that's me." In this process of physical conversion, he becomes a "subject" because of the recognition that the hail or the call was "really" addressed to him, and that it was really he who was hailed and not someone else.

The Althusserean model of interpellation is used by the single, unified Repressive State Apparatus (RSA) that is usually accompanied by the multiple, disunited Ideological State Apparatuses (ISAs). The RSA that consists of the government, the administration, the army, the judiciary and the prison system is also, in Buchanan's words, "known in contemporay political discourse as 'hard power', i.e. a form of power that operates [...] primarily by means of mental and physical coercion and violence (latent and actual)" (407). The ISAs that comprise mostly semi-autonomous, private or non-governmental organizations such as churches, public or private educational institutions, the political system or parties, trade unions, the media, the family and the cultural things are understood, in Buchanan's words, "in contemporary political discourse as 'soft power', i.e. the form of power that operates by means of ideological persuasion

[...]"(242). Althusser believes that any form of government, be it repressive and violent or democratic and liberal, requires ideology to run smoothly. Arguing from a Maoist position, he says that power must come out of the barrel of a gun, must be made definite and clear in the minds of individuals. Through the separation of the state from the apparatuses the state requires for its maintenance, Althusser implies that revolutionaries need to capture power and to control the apparatuses of power at the same time. Thus, the Althusseran model is used by institutional apparatuses to bring individual's imaginary notion of the self and society into a "specific" form of societal reality and subjectivity. This process of subjectification that is attained in and through subjection only accords the person the status of the social subject. This is how people come to recognize, consider themselves, and to feel and think that an identity is the one which fits them.

Althusser claims that "The existence of ideology and the hailing or interpellation of individuals as subjects are one and the same thing" (131). For him, a child before its birth is "always-already a subject, appointed as a subject in and by the specific familial ideological configuration in which it is expected once it has been conceived"(132). The configurations or forms of family ideology are paternal, maternal, conjugal, fraternal and sororal. Althusser stresses the key role played by the family that hails or addresses individuals before they are born. Despite the sharp differentiation between the addresser (the speaking subject) and the addressed (the spoken subject) in the Althusserean scheme, they are, however, inter-linked for the simple reason that the latter is constituted only through the subject of speech by the former. This model shows that there is always a link between the personal and the social, and that sociocultural structures work to recruit people into identities.

The postmodern critics develop their theory of "identity" by appropriating the deconstructionist notion of indeterminacy of language and meaning. This needs further clarification. Saussurean scheme (discussed above) is critiqued by the Post-structuralist philosopher Jacques Derrida who opposes the notion of absoluteness and irreducibility in the differences between the signifier and the signified, since it entails the presence of "the transcendental or the original signified." The central or transcendental signified is the autonomous and final concept that is independent of a given signifying system it seeks to articulate and is incapable of relating beyond itself to any other term. Saussure invokes Western metaphysical oppositionist scheme that privileges the signified (thought, concept or spirit) over the signifier (form, substance or matter). Derrida argues that every signified is replaceable, substitutable, and is present within the system it tries to determine. The signifieds derive their meanings and values from its location within a larger structure that precedes it. Hence there is no essence. Everything has structurality. He writes, "The substitute does not substitute itself for anything which has somehow existed before it. Henceforth, it was necessary to begin thinking that there was no center .[...] in the absence of a center or origin, everything became discourse [...] that is to say, a system in which the central signified, the original or transcendental signified, is never absolutely present outside a system of differences. The absence of the transcendental signified extends the domain and play of signification infinitely" (*Writing and Difference* 280). Thus, every signified commutes for another and operates in turn as a signifier in a perpetual play of signification. In this process of supplementarity, the signifier is proliferated out of the signified. Meaning gets slipped or displaced from one term to another and tends eternally to be indeterminate. The human subject is caught in the webs of significations, since the "subject" and "signification" interdependently yet differentially always keep shifting and are unstable.

Using this notion of Derrida's deconstruction, the

postmodern critics of "identity" argue, "the self - as a unified, stable, and knowable entity existing prior to or outside language - is merely a fiction of language, an effect of discourse" (Moya 6). Thus, everything is always already there as "construction" of language of people, society and culture. Identity is always heterogeneous, fractured. This is the notion of anti-essentialism, of constructionism.

This linguistic, constructionist position of identity has been viewed psychoanalytically with the emphasis on "the unconscious" by the French psychologist Jacques Lacan who shares and revises as well some ideas of the Austrian psychoanalyst Sigmund Freud. Freud rejects the Cartesian notion of "awareness" or "the conscious" only constituting the "mind" by focussing on "the unconscious"that is defined as that part of the mind which is latent, hidden from and inaccessible to the conscious mind but which affects behaviour, emotions, etc.

The notion of the unconscious needs further explanation. A child is not allowed to do or to have all the things he or she needs or wants, and in the process, represses his or her feelings and desires. These suppressed or repressed materials pass into the unconscious and are manifested in later life through fears, memories, wishes, dreams and Freudian slips (the word uttered is not the word intended). These in turn often influence the adult human "identity" that is constituted by the conflation of the pastness (the unconscious feelings) of childhood experience and the rational (conscious) present. This suggests fluid, incoherent and changing nature of identity. This is the earlier Freud who was very close to constructionism. The "divide" between the conscious and the unconscious through the repression barrier is popularly known as the descriptive or "topographic model" that was revised later by Freud. The revised model is called "ego-psychology" whereby the ego becomes both part of the unconscious ("id") and the conscious ("super-ego") as well. Ego-psychology seeks to project the ego, or subject as an unbroken, coherent entity and thereby contradicts the earlier Freud who believes in the divide. This is the later Freud who was an essentialist.

Freud's theory of the Oedipus complex draws attention to the fact that the major concern of psychoanalysis is sex, sexuality and gender. It is framed from the story of the legendary Greek king, Oedipus who unknowingly killed his father and married his mother. The theory is about the complex of emotions aroused "naturally" in a young (male) child, typically around the age of four, by an unconscious sexual desire for the mother and by a wish to eliminate the father so as to take his (father's) place. Being unable to exclude his father, the child takes father's identity into himself and thereby both loves and hates his father even as he both desires and resents his mother. This initial hostile bisexuality of the child diminishes as his identification with the image of the parent of the same sex continues to grow till it effects a removal of his father by incorporation of his father in himself. The child admires his father even though his affection for the mother continues. The female child marked by the absence of a penis, according to Freud, feels "lack" or "castrated," even though her first love object is the mother who is in due course perceived as not only deficient herself but as the cause of the daughter's deficiency. Subsequently she views the entire female sex in this light. For this reason, she rejects her mother and turns towards her father who becomes the central figure in her psychic register. This replacement of one parent by the other without identification with the same sex causes violent interruptions in daughter's erotic life that remains heterosexual, procreative and patriarchal. This is the female Oedipus complex.

These theories have raised controversies, since as Kaja Silverman notes, "anatomy only acquires meaning and value as the consequence of intense cultural mediation" (142). However, in the Freudian scheme, children are sexual and develop psycho-sexually. It implies that both gender and sexuality are crucial to the understanding of identity. Peoples' sense of who they are is prominently associated with their awareness of their identities as men or as women. Freud's naturalist project of the Oedipus complex represents essentialism, universalism and foundationalism. In other words, the Freudian subject has a pre-given identity.

Freud's ideas are reread by Lacan who does not subscribe to the "ego-psychology" of the later Freud. Lacan argues in favour of the topographic model of the earlier Freud. For him, the "I" or ego or subject is always "split" within itself and is constituted by a conscious, knowable mind and by an unconscious, unknowable series of forces and drives. The unconscious that is not "recognized" by the subject as an aspect of itself is the Other. It is experienced by the subject as the other from itself. The subject's own desire is projected on to the Other which in turn sees itself in the subject. The subject does not know that its own unconsciousness is a part of itself and hence "misrecognizes" its own unconsciousness as the Other. Consequently, it fails to recognize that it desires what the Other desires. That is why, as Francoise Meltzer puts it, "Lacan's famous maxim is that 'the unconscious is the discourse of the Other.'[...] unconsciousness emerges as otherness within consciousness" (158). The dialectic of the conscious/unconscious has been paralleled with the subject/Other. Of course, in the Oedipal sense the father is the real Other. However, the Lacanian father, unlike the Freudian one, is not natural but normative. It is "the 'Name-of-the-Father,' rather than the biological father *per se*" (Fuss 7). The Name-of-the-Father is the paternal signifier. In this context, it is also important to note that for Lacan, the "phallus" is a representational symbol and "not" an anatomical organ, "not a fantasy, not an object, and most especially not an organ (the penis or the clitoris) [...]. The phallus is instead a *signifier*, [...] is *prior* to the penis; [...] is the privileged mark through which both sexes accede to sexual identity by a recognition and acceptance of castration" (Fuss 8). Identity of the Lacanian subject is constructed through language, symbol and metaphor.

The Lacanian subject is also constituted by a "lack." The Lacanian theory of the subject defined by lack has three registers: the "real," the "imaginary" and the "symbolic." The "real" that fails to differentiate sexes (male or female) in terms of "signification" begins from the moment of zygote formation within the womb till the separation of the child from the mother at birth. The "real" by being subject to sex lacks the "primordial" notion of living being as the androgynous whole. This is the first lack. Thus, the primordial (always the pre-Oedipal) psychological wholeness is a fantasy that is intermittently ruptured by a series of lacks that spell anxiety. The second lack occurs in the subject after birth when its body is materially and culturally prepared for the sexual differentiation. The mouth, the anus, the penis and the vagina of the child are most frequently taken care of by the mother who in the process territorializes, defines and inscribes the body and the erotic zones of the baby. The third lack starts between the ages of six months and eighteen months of the subject when it enters the "imaginary" or "mirror stage." It is a stage of identification and duality, of the subject's self and the other. The subject lacks the coherence of its own reflection in the mirror. The mirror image of the subject is its lateral inversion that it recognizes to be its own self. This is mis-recognition. The subject's perception of objects is structured by and vacillates between the two extremes or binary oppositions such as love and hate. This points to the self-alienation of the subject who knows itself through an external image. The fourth lack is shown in the "symbolic" order that marks the subject's access to "language" and the Oedipal complex. In this symbolic register only, the subject learns the notion of "lack," of "the Other," and brings the unconscious into existence. The discourse of the Other within which the subject's identity is formed takes place in this symbolic order. As Fuss puts it, "the Symbolic represents the order of language which permits the child entry into subjectivity, into the realm of speech, law, and sociality. The Imaginary signifies the mother-child dyad which the Symbolic interrupts through the agency of the paternal function – the 'Name-of-the-Father,' [...]" (7). For Lacan, the Oedipus complex is also symbolic. However, all these stages are not free from cultural intervention that contributes significantly to the making of the identity of the child.

The Lacanian "lack" then is purely sexual in definition. Lack ('manque') in turn engenders or is experienced as "desire" which animals (except their biological need) do not experience psychologically. This desire in the unconscious is, in the Freudian sense, forever displaced (distorted) and disguised as something else (called the state of repression) and in the process causes tension (displeasure) that seeks hydraulically (involuntarily) release into consciousness to achieve the "stasis" or pleasure resulting in the absence (stoppage) of desire. After the stasis is attained, a "gap" is produced. The unconscious reveals itself in laying stress on filling the "gap" that is felt by the subject as a lack in him or her. This lack in turn generates desire in the subject, and desire always remains unfulfilled.

Displacing the classical humanist subject in favour of linguistic production of the subject, Lacan says that the unconscious is structured like a language. The unconscious is formed in the same manner as the subject's inborn ability for language. The innate structures in the mind for the making of an unconscious and for language acquisition are the same. That is why the subject is unaware of the signifying processes. To explain this, Lacan combines the Saussurean concept of a linguistic sign as the union of the signifier and the signified with the Russian-born American linguist Roman Jakobson's idea of "metaphor" (a word-for-word substitution based semantically on the notion of similarity) and "metonymy" (a word-to-word displacement based syntactically on the principle of contiguity). The signifier is the unconscious and the signified the conscious. Lacan privileges the signifier over the signified. Metaphor and metonymy, for Lacan, are what Francoise Meltzer calls "the rhetoric of the unconscious" (159). Meltzer writes:

> Metonymy [...] is a chain of signifiers that are horizontal, [...] is the signifier of desire [...]. What is desired is always displaced, always deferred, and reappears endlessly in another guise. Desire, in other words, is the signifier that never changes [...]. In spite of its apparent difference of meaning (the signifieds) in each case, each signifier in this chain has in fact the same meaning as the one before it: the lack which spells desire. Metaphor, on the other hand, is a vertical, non-contiguous structure, and is a system of substitution rather than displacement. For Lacan, [...] this can be shown by saying that one signifier can substitute as the signified for another signifier. (160)

Thus, in this Lacanian model, unfulfillable unconscious desire marked as and by "lack" is eternally displaced (transformed) or substituted for, thereby constituting a chain of signifiers, a chain that like the unconscious perpetually leaves its own traces. Thus, the Lacanian subject is fragmented both linguistically and unconsciously. It also suggests that there is, as Ernesto Laclau puts it, "a lack at the root of any identity; one needs to identify with some one because there is an originary and insurmountable lack of identity" (3). By extending the naturalist Freudian model through the interconnections between psychoanalysis on the one hand and linguistic and anthropological semiotics on the other, the Lacanian model synthesizes subject, signifier and culture and thereby argues for subject positions or multiple and mobile identities. The Lacanian identity is always alienated, fictitious, contingent and provisional. Most importantly, as Fuss puts it, "The Lacanian subject is a sexed subject first and last" (10).

This linguistic-cum-psychoanalytic reductionism of postmodern identity as against the nonreductionist universal paradigm of the Cartesian identity known through the "dualism" expressed as the conscious mind controlling the body has triggered polarization between constructionism and essentialism that, however, overlap and converge when the question of "the body" that a person inhabits emerges. Essentialists would argue that the body is "natural," "pre-" or "a-" social and is always out there as the "real" thing. The constructionist position is that the body is always already socioculturally created. Now how can the hunger, thirst, pain, suffering, palpable pathological signs, illness and death of the body be accounted for, even though they are understood in a socially determined manner? What is more immediately and inseparably linked to the subject than the experience of its own body that is obviously inaccessible in its exactness to the social others? Is it possible to have the sociocultural understanding of the subject's experience even prior to the subject's knowledge of it? After all, identity is not apprehended in abstraction but in a given spatiotemporal location. As Madan Sarup argues, "any study of identity must be localised in space and time. [...] the study of identity must be based on something called 'evidence' and we must be aware of our methods of perception" (15). The body is the space, time and evidence of identity. As Paul Ricoeur would write, "Possessing bodies is precisely what persons do indeed do, or rather what they actually are" (33). However, "developing" a particular kind of body (for example, through gendering, sexualizing, racializing, politicizing, plastic surgery, bodybuilding, boxing, etc.) is social. This argument makes a case for the compromise between the arbitrary notion of essentialism and the deterministic project of constructionism. This compromise is perhaps at the root of Satya P. Mohanty's postpositivist realist theory of identity, a theory which is practised by some critics who insist that, as Paula M.L.Moya in her essay "Postmodernism, 'Realism,' and the Politics of Identity: Cherrie Moraga and Chicana Feminism" sums up:

> we acknowledge and interrogate the consequences - social, political, economic, and epistemic – of social location. To do this, we must first acknowledge the reality of those social categories (race, class, gender, and sexuality) that together make up an individual's social location. We do not need to see these categories as uncontestable or absolutely fixed to acknowledge their ontological status. We do, however, need to recognize that they have real material effects and that their effects are systematic rather than accidental. A realist theory of identity understands that while identities are not fixed, neither are they random. There is a nonarbitrary limit to the range of identities we can plausibly 'construct' or 'choose' for any individual in a given society. (87)

Identity requires "labelling" either by the subject itself or by the collectivities such as the society, culture and nation for its manifestation. The label in turn forms the "categorization" theory that places identity in a class or division. When the most typical, conventional or common characteristic of the category is represented in an exaggerated, oversimplified manner it is called "stereotype" whereby a person or thing conforms to an unjustifiably fixed or standardized mental picture. Here power comes into play in order to be dominant and hegemonic, since categorization entails inclusion of some people by exclusion of others. Exclusion then is justified through "stigma" that aims at demeaning, discrediting or disgracing either the categorized (the "in-group" or "us") or the noncategorized (the "out-group" or "them"). This classification theory also generates a tendency for people or a person of a particular religion, race, social background, gender, sexuality,etc., to form exclusive political alliances, to engage with politics founded on the exclusive sense of group or personal identity, moving away from traditional broad-based party politics. For example, someone is classified as a female, as a gay, as a Black, as a person living with AIDS. This tendency is known as "identity politics."

Hence categorization is both descriptive and prescriptive (normative), thereby encouraging discrimination and hierarchy. "Sex" and "gender" through which everyone is categorized as either a "male" or a "female" and is characteristically stereotyped as either the "masculine" or the "feminine" are the most basic and controversial examples, needing further discussion particularly in the context of the present study concerning HIV/AIDS.

Conventionally, sex and gender are understood as the same things or terms meaning the states of being males or females. They are regarded as biological and are defined in terms of the anatomical organs that signify men and women. However, in social sciences though "sex" is understood as a natural, biological given, the term "gender" refers to the social and cultural practices or performances that produce sexed bodies. Social practices such as wearing of clothes that present gender hints even as they hide genitalia and hence the bodily evidence can be one instance. Likewise at the genetic level, sometimes it is possible to have two X chromosomes and one Y chromosome instead of either only two X chromosomes (for women) or one X and one Y chromosome (for men), even though chromosomal category is taken for granted. Eunuchs and hermaphrodites do not belong to the gender identity category because of their gender incoherence. Even a child is groomed domestically, educationally or whatever to imbibe feminine or masculine traits by the gender-appropriate behaviours of a society and a culture. The children learn to categorize themselves as boys or girls between two and three years of age. Law and the mass media also inform people to categorize themselves. Therefore gender is constructed and used. The cultural apparatus genders a person.

However, men and women differ from each other in the materiality of their bodies, particularly in the menstruating and reproductive capability of "most" (not all) women of certain age, a capability that men do not have. At this point poststructuralists argue, "in seeking to map and catalogue these differences, to order them along certain axes, to describe the objective 'reality' of bodies, the descriptor will inevitably impose particular understandings and values to construct a particular version of what is described" (Sheldon 21).

In this sociological, constructionist perspective, gender is cultural causing sex/gender binarism. This binarism is challenged by the French philosopher Michel Foucault who in *The History of Sexuality* observes, "Sexuality must not be thought of as a kind of natural given [...]. It is the name that can be given to a historical construct [...]" (105). Sexuality is not the trans-historical or pre-cultural quality of the body. Following Foucault, Judith Butler in *Bodies that Matter* also argues, "The category of 'sex' is, from the start, normative; [...] a 'regulatory ideal' [...] that produces the bodies it governs, that is, whose regulatory force is made clear as a kind of productive power, the power to produce – demarcate, circulate, differentiate – the bodies it controls [...]. In other words, 'sex' is an ideal construct which is forcibly materialized through time" (1). The normativization of sex seeks to impose certain values to serve and maintain the interest of the heterosexual imperative and thereby rules out the materiality of the body. Thus, sex like gender is also culturally constructed. The body is constructed through language, through discourse, since "there is no reference to a pure body which is not at the same time a further formation of that body" (*Bodies* 10). Thus, "the body" understood through social mediation is disembodied, and "identities" in relation to the bodies are always already gendered, sexualized.

This argument is reinforced by Butler's notion of performativity. Butler draws on Nietzsche's idea that "there is no 'being' behind doing, effecting, becoming; 'the doer' is merely a fiction added to the deed - the deed is everything" (45). She argues that gender is "performative." Blurring the distinction between gender and sex, she argues in *Gender Trouble* that "There is no gender identity behind the expressions of gender; that identity is performatively constituted by the very 'expressions' that are said to be its results" (25). In her view sex itself is gendered by performance. Thus, the performance of gender can cause subversion of essential and dominant notions of gendered and sexed identities such as male or female, gay and lesbian or straight. The queer theorist Elizabeth Grosz privileges sex over gender by arguing that sex itself and bodies themselves are unstable. Therefore, she pleads, "what anybody is capable of doing is well beyond the tolerance of any given culture" (qtd. in Milner and Browitt 138). For her, all bodies being always necessarily the objects and subjects of attitudes and judgments are sites of "mediations" or "exchanges" between the biological (private) and the cultural (public), the psychological and the social. However, Grosz like Butler, does not believe in the "pure" materiality of the body. The anti-essentialist and disunited notions of sexuality and identity are further connected to "fetishism" by Thomas Yingling who argues that "fetishism [...] has been defined in psychoanalysis [...] as the denial of lack. All identity is fetishistic in that it is structured on the denial of self-difference and absence; identity, that is, cannot occur except through fundamental (and generative) misrecognitions" (112). The "reality" of sexuality and identity is a fantasy.

"Sexual identity" of a human being is ,therefore, structured out of the densely connected groups of already existing different forms of knowledge, power, desire and pleasure centering on bodies. Bodies are continually shaped by the "panoptic" gaze of both imagined and real interpretative communities and are shown and seen as the political things. As Foucault in *Discipline and Punish* describes, "The body is directly involved in a political field; power relations have an immediate hold upon it; they invest it, train it, torture it, force it to carry out tasks, to perform ceremonies and to emit signs" (25). He suggests that systems of surveillance - surveillance that is either actually existing or imagined to be existing - shape and discipline the body. Andrew Edgar in his article "body" rightly sums up, "Analysis of the body can therefore increasingly see it as a product of social constraint and construction [...], or of the languages and discourses within which it is discussed and analysed (as for example, in the languages of medical science, psychiatry, or criminology)" (47).

However, feminists, sociologists and philosophers are embodied subjects themselves. They therefore must not, according to the Canadian feminist philosopher Susan Wendell, "confuse the lived reality of bodies with cultural discourse about and representations of bodies [...]. I do not think my body is a cultural representation, although I recognize that my experience of it is both highly interpreted and very influenced by cultural (including medical) representations. Moreover, [...] it would be cruel, as well as a distortion of people's lives, to [...] simply [...] recognize that human bodies and their varied conditions are both changeable and highly interpreted" (44). As an ME (chronic fatigue and depression syndrome) patient herself, she realizes that the constructionist position of the body erases or ignores the everyday, practical and experienced limitations of people's disabilities.

In a postpositivist realist mode S. Williams and G. Bendelow plead that sociology should theorize "not so much *about* bodies [...] but *from* bodies as *lived* entities [...]. Social institutions and discursive practices cannot be understood apart from the real lived experiences and actions of embodied human beings across time and space. Social theory must therefore be rooted in the problems of human embodiment" (209). This is best realized, or illustrated through the impaired, disabled and diseased bodies. As Carol Thomas puts it, "Those of us who live with marked impairments know that the body is 'real' however thoroughly it is culturally represented and positioned" (77). Sociology of disease, disability and pain therefore needs to be able to negotiate the real materiality of bodies with the interpretative communities around bodies.

The body is neither natural nor social. The fact remains that people live in their bodies that serve multiple (often ambiguous) purposes, conceal their "selfhood" projected always as "otherness." As Paul Ricouer points out, "the selfhood of oneself implies otherness to such an intimate degree that one cannot be thought of without the other, that instead one passes into the other [...]" (3). Bodies can be mothers, fathers, children, drag queens, masters, slaves, gays, blacks, whites, politicians, citizens and so on. Coupled with the "experiences" of these bodies in constantly "changing" times and locations, multiple and perhaps uncertain (work-related and income-related, for example) identities will continue to emerge. These identities constituted through experiences will then have material, epistemic and political effects. That is why bodies as the significant constitutive domain of identities matter. And identities, as Paula M. L. Moya with an ethical aim adds, "are often assumed or chosen for complex subjective reasons that can be objectively evaluated" (Introduction 9). In course of evaluation, the pros and cons of the statuses of identities can be unprejudicedly understood so as to effect transformation, acceptance or dismantlement of those factors (structures, agencies or subjectivities) that have produced them.

IV

With this ethical objective, identity-related multiperspectival questions that the disease (HIV/AIDS) discourse has very fiercely raised will be examined. In the first two sections of this chapter, linguistic representations of HIV/AIDS through different "labels" that have been given to the virus and through metaphors have been discussed. The "impact" of such representation on the developing or finding of identity of the subject will be analyzed in the light of the third section's apparently digressive but highly contextual discussion on the question of identity. Drawing from the Lacanian notion of the subject, it can be argued that "representation", such as above-mentioned disease labels and metaphors, at the "psychological" level intensifies the "innate" sense of denial or shame in the mind of the diseased in regard to the acceptance of disease.

At the mental level, it is usually seen that even though disease is a common experience, people often initially refuse to acknowledge the presence of illness in their own bodies up to the stage of public or social manifestation. The cause for this irrepressible impulse for denial is stated to be phobic. "Denial" can be understood as fear of being associated with illness. The genesis of denial lies, as Manfred Bleuler points out, in "our own prejudiced thinking. We conceive ourselves, our personalities, and our own egos as being steady and firm. The fact that we could disintegrate [...] is a monstrous, uncanny concept" (8). This "prejudiced thinking" of one's own steadiness or firmness and non-disintegration is the fantasy of the self or the subject. This deep-rooted fantasy of the self denies the sense of its own breakdown and as a result, is externalized, projected in the form of a persona that is a fiction of the self as shown to or perceived by others. This persona produced by denial is the misrecognized or the fictitious "other," the subject's unrecognized, repressed unconscious in a Lacanian sense. As has been discussed earlier, psychoanalysis shows that selfhood is formed through a succession of identifications. By the psychological process of identification, the subject "assimilates an aspect, property, or attribute of the other and is transformed, wholly or partially, after the model the other provides" (Laplanche and Pontalis 205).

However, the process of identifying, according to Simon Watney, "operates in two modes: the transitive one of identifying the self in relation to the *difference* of the other, and the reflexive one of identifying the self in a relation of *resemblance* to the other" (*Practices* 52). The self in disease initially both transitively and reflexively relates itself to the "difference" of and the "resemblance" to the other even as it compares the material effects of illness on it with its "own prejudiced thinking" or fantasy about its non-integration. Consequently, it is filled with fear of being stigmatized, a fear that is then expressed as denial only to avoid social visibility of its diseased state. This denial is an aspect of the definition of "selfhood" in the context of illness. This sense gets strengthened by its response to disease labels and metaphors given above. This is in one register.

However, in another register this denial does not prolong as the subject being entirely affected both in the body and in the mind by disease acquires a separate identity. The diseased subject starts defining itself against the other, since the latter differs from and hence threatens the separateness of the former. It recognizes that it is what the other is not. Thus, it becomes hostile to the other and feels insecure. To overcome the sense of insecurity concealed in the sense of difference, the subject seeks its oneness with the social through "self-categorization." In the process, it labels itself by identifying itself with the social and cultural categories or tropes that always, in the Althussrean sense, interpellate or hail the individual. The mental and physical states of being and becoming ill are always seen through the social projection of the ill by the sick. This mode of construction of one's own sense of oneself as "patient" is what Sander L. Gilman calls "self-stereotyping" (6).

This self-standardizing then can be either denied or affirmed, since the cultural categorization is a site of projection of different sense of the self. This reaction depends on how the experiencing subject identifies its own feeling with the determined or imagined community experiences, of which it is already ascribed to be a part. Absolute failure to internalize or identify might result in the production of "new" category or identity. This is associated with the "newness" of experience. For example, the new category "people living with AIDS" refers to, as Thomas Yingling describes his own experience of the disease, " non-subjects, people for whom the mirroring illusions of discourse are broken: the host body in this case continually reminds its subject - with every glance in the mirror - of the distance between the 'I' and its lesions [...]. The struggle in living with AIDS is to produce [...] a new identity, new codification and damming of the flow of desire [...] in the body [...]" (16). The HIV-positive subject experiences a state of desirelessness. There is alienation of a subject from a body. The impossibility of speaking the condition of loss being written into (and onto) the body is what the diseased person experiences. Yingling writes, "So it is not desire that is in question, but identity: the whole problem of a disappearing body, of a body quite literally shitting itself away. That is AIDS" (16).

The above two registers show that the impact of "articulation" or representation of disease through and in language problematizes the notion of illness. Any articulation is an "ethical" question, since it tends to hierarchize by being judgmental. To acknowledge is to differ, assort and hence isolate. To accept the ill is to classify and isolate patients thought to be contagious or infectious. This "moral" model of disease also causes balkanization of the identity of the sick. For example, as Edward Albert has shown, "Three categories of people with AIDS can be documented: the innocent, the suspect, and the guilty" (174). The blameless or the innocent in the context of HIV/AIDS are those who contract the disease without indulging in any risk practice and without any "fault" of their own, such as the newborn, haemophiliacs, surgery patients, thalassemics, people subjected to religious rites of physical incision such as the tattooed, the circumcised and to sexual violence like rape, etc. The suspect are those (for instance, bisexuals) who hide their promiscuous/deviant lifestyle to medical professionals because of stigma, engage in unsafe sex and thereby contract and spread the disease. The guilty are seen as those (such as homosexuals or drug users or prostitutes or infected blood donors) who, despite their knowledge of themselves being at risk, engage in anonymous, kinky unsafe sex or drug use to spread the disease. Sometimes all kinds of "disfigurements" (for example, structural alterations or physical deformities) and "dissolutions" caused by disease are chosen as the parameters to organize the identity of the diseased subject. This practice is based on, in Sontag's words, "aesthetic judgements about the beautiful and the ugly, the clean and the unclean, the familiar and the alien or uncanny" (41). The aesthetic category is occasionally juxtaposed with the moral class. This moral system often stigmatizes, degrades one's status and thereby transforms individual's status.

However, this shows that the "ethical" is enmeshed and embedded in "politics" suggesting strategies or tactics in activities. This also reveals that articulation or representation in itself is "political" in its potential to seek privilege or status and "power" that are subsequently reified as authorities, like the crowned heads, the religious heads, and the heads of families, groups, communities, institutions, states, nations, etc. Power is inherently dominant, hegemonic and hence authoritative and is, at the same time, innately capable of being resisted. In the light of this "political" model, disease is viewed as something that exceeds its metaphoric significance. Allan M. Brandt remarks, "[...] disease is more than a metaphor. These 'social constructions' are more than merely metaphors. They have very real sociopolitical implications" (148).

The "political" implication of disease can be best understood in Mary Douglas's theory of contagion and accusation. Inquiring politically into "disease" as an effective resource for maintaining hegemony or authority, Douglas considers "accusations" of illness. Any community engaged in power struggle, in rejection and assertion of authority within and without its boundary has used "disease" as an "accusation." By reading accusation simultaneously into witchcraft and leprosy, Douglas highlights the hidden potential of infectious diseases to exclude certain categories of people. The victim, the accuser and the accused involved in accusations keep changing their positions from time to time as per their targets to maintain balance of power in different cultural regimes. The fear of being dominated by a certain group is countered by the use of "disease" (e.g. HIV/AIDS) that is in this context regarded as an effective tool. Douglas's theory posits a social hierarchy comprising both "the central community"representing the dominant class and the three "peripheries" ("Dissenting Enclave," "Individualist" and "Isolate") symbolizing the marginal categories. The former always engages in controlling the latter that, in turn, resist: "When it comes to a particular disease, the existing attempts on the part of the central community to segregate itself and control its borders have their effect on others. The established theory has to do battle with alternative theories developed to prevent the community from tightening its control over its periphery" (Douglas 112). Hence accusation or blame on the one hand and activism or resistance on the other go hand in hand.

In Douglas's model, epidemics provide occasions for certain "group ideologies" to become hegemonic. They are exploited to promote, protect and safeguard the interests of status or power within an organization, and in doing so influence the state, government or public affairs. Hence, illness becomes "political." This accusation model as normative and regulatory apparatus can be seen, for instance, in the nationalist construction of foreign origin theory of illness, a theory that emanates from the feeling that "national identity requires an ideal conception of the body and a rejection of accommodation to Otherness" (Yingling 25). The Otherness refers to physical, moral and sexual diseases. To project itself as the ideal and uncontaminated land, a nation depicts foreigners as vectors or carriers of illnesses. As Sontag observes, "Epidemics of particularly dreaded illnesses always provoke an outcry against leniency or tolerance - now identified as [...] unhealthiness. Demands are made to subject people to 'tests,' to isolate the ill and those suspected of being ill or of transmitting illness, and to erect barriers against the real or imaginary contamination of foreigners" (80). This promotes and intensifies xenophobia. This results in nativists's demand for surveillance and, sometimes, for deportation of and, if necessary, complete ban on immigrants, even though there are lab evidences of decreased incidence of disease.

Disease thus inculpates some both figurally and literally and in so doing exculpates others. This political implication is also seen in the epidemiological and the public health practices, such as screening, testing, case reporting and contact tracing for certain infectious, communicable and contagious diseases, the quarantine and isolation of the infected, and disease surveillance, control and prevention. In the political form of disease, the identity of the diseased is determined, as Allan M.

Brandt rightly points out, by "the pervasive fear of contagion, concerns about casual transmission, the stigmatization of victims, the conflicts between public health and civil liberties and the search for magic bullets" (163).

Questing for "magic bullets" being a metaphor for inexplicably surprising treatment and cure in the epidemic condition of disease, the government authorities and the mass media circulate figurative categorizations with such force and frequency as to cause "panic" that is accepted to be logical. This situation is very aptly described by Linda Singer as "a panic logic which seeks immediate and dramatic responses to the situation at hand" (28). This epidemic logic, as Singer very cogently argues, is structured along contradictions, proliferates what it seeks to contain, produces what it regulates, revives perpetually an anxiety of contagion that it seeks to control. The effects of this logic induced by metaphors are far-reaching. It constructs public "phobia" or, as Sontag feels, "fears of easy contagion and bizarre fantasies of transmission [...] in public places" (27). Venereal diseases, for instance, inspire fears of transmission through nonvenereal means such as transmission through sharing drinking cups, glasses, pens, pencils, toothbrushes, towels, beds, public toilet seats and so on. Hence, one is, as John Donne observes, "preafflicted, superafflicted with [...] apprehensions of Sicknes, before we can cal it a sicknes; [...] we are tormented with sicknes and cannot stay till the torment come, but preapprehensions and presages, prophecy those torments, which induce that death before either come; and our dissolution is conceived in these first changes, quickened in the sicknes itselfe, and borne in death, which beares date from these first changes" (417-18). Donne talks about how the processes of "dissolution" and "death" of the sick are constructed out of "apprehensions of Sicknes." This panic also causes the diseased to feel abandoned, since the feared infectiousness of the disease prevents people from visiting them. The patient thus suffers more through the arousal of fear of stigmatization and abandonment than through the awareness of suffering from disease.

The "spoiling" of identity of the diseased is further complicated by the production of ideologically chosen terms that are complicit in the panic logic. These terms are carefully framed to maintain leadership or rulership status by communal or national regimes, since any "ideology" required to rule or to generate consent to be ruled must formulate its own vocabularies. These vocabularies circulate as "keywords" that can be identified as conveying, to use Raymond Williams's words, "not resolution but perhaps, at times, just that extra edge of consciousness. In a social history in which many crucial meanings have been shaped by a dominant class, and by particular professions operating to a large extent within its terms, the sense of edge is accurate. This is not a neutral review of meanings" (24).

Key vocabularies that are the products of ideological needs indubitably have the "edge,"superiority or advantage that can produce differentiation, dominance, challenges and responses at the same time. These, despite the impossibility to delink them from their past implications (specifically social, historical and linguistic ones) that, as always, integrate the problems of meanings and relationships, are sometimes used in a new way to generate hegemony. Disease metaphor such as "the alien" or "the foreign" for risk-group, for example, is always used for the colonized by the colonizers in colonial discourse. As Sontag has pointed out, "Part of the centuries-old conception of Europe as a privileged cultural entity is that it is a place which is colonized by lethal diseases coming from elsewhere. Europe is assumed to be by rights free of disease" (50). Corollarily, the developing countries are seen as the diseased others by the industrial nations of the West. In the US, according to Yingling, "the American feeling for the body inscribes disease as foreign and allows AIDS to be read therefore as anti-American" (25). This is why Americans wilfully believe the disease to be of Third World or African origin, since Africans are presumed to be hypersexual, practise anal sex as a form of birth control, have no sense of health and hygiene, and have very limited access to medical knowledge and care.

HIV/AIDS discourse including its pedagogics since its genesis has frequently developed and used certain AIDS-related keywords that are intended to foster public awareness of the need for both, according to Cindy Patton, "information and [...] attitude change"(*Inventing* 113). These keywords in their different stages of development show that, as Jan Zita Grover points out, "AIDS is not simply a physical malady; it is also an artifact of social and sexual transgression, violated taboo, fractured identity - political and personal projections. Its keywords [...] are primarily the property of the powerful" (18). They are GRID, gay/ homosexual community, AIDS Test, lesbian, bisexual, carrier/spread, risk group, victim, PWA (Person with AIDS)/PLWA (People living with AIDS), general population/heterosexual community, prostitute, risk practice, promiscuity/safe sex, condone, family and Just Say No.

These key terms need close examination especially in consideration of the focus of this chapter, since they will reveal the politics of HIV/AIDS and identity as well in the US. The acronym GRID (gay-related immune deficiency) was initially coined by some scientists in the US in January 1982 for what is now known as HIV/AIDS, which was then primarily seen as a "gay male disease" focussing on the "male homosexuality" as a pathological thing. This radically problematized the very notion of "sexual identity."

The same-sex desires, pleasures and social bondings, as Foucault has shown in his *The History of Sexuality*, were viewed in male-centered patriarchy as natural and sacred things in ancient Greek society. These were replaced by "marriage" and "wife" only in transition from ancient

Greece to ancient Rome during the first two centuries AD. "Heterosexuality" since then has been normativised as the "natural" and compulsory thing in direct opposition to "homosexuality" that has been denaturalized, and associated with fear and hatred known as "homophobia." As Sedgwick observes, "'obligatory heterosexuality' is built into male-dominated kinship systems [...]" (3). She also notes, "[...] homophobia is a *necessary* consequence of such patriarchal institutions as heterosexual marriage" (3). She further suggests that patriarchy structurally includes and therefore requires homophobia.

"Heterosexuality" stands for the privileging of the procreative, the family over the erotic. Hence, "nongenerative" homosexuals without having any sexual and family constraints are always considered against the grain, against the canon of mandatory heterosexism and are viewed as "perverts" or "deviants." The term GRID fiercely raised questions about the biological or natural, social and cultural positions of "sex," "gender," "sexuality" and "subjectivity" that are the crucial features of "identity." Following the claims of Foucault, Butler and Grosz that sex and gender are not pre-social but social and cultural constructs, it may be argued that genderwise "male" socioculturally constructed by the penis is always seen as presiding over "female" recognized by the vagina. In terms of sexuality defined either by its "orientation" or by its "preference," heterosexuality is constructed and perceived as predominating over homosexuality and lesbianism that are always marginalized to the point of making them inconspicuous. As Tamsin Wilton puts it, "a body which has a vagina and uterus is understood as *for* penetration (and by implication, impregnation) by a penis, while a body which has a penis is understood as *for* penetrating (and impregnating) a vagina/uterus. The meaning of the body (perceived as 'sexed') is a sexual/erotic one [...]" (15).

Concerning subjectivity, it is "the masculine" that is privileged, imitated, performed and hence negotiated both at individual and national levels for maturity, production, reproduction and health. The masculine subject is a disembodied one free from suffering. The male body might suffer, but the male spirit transcends it. As against certain historical principles of feminism, any notion of the subject is, as Yingling notes, "always already masculine [...]" (25). This is the paradigmatic and socially desirable notion of hetero-patriarchal system.

Thus, the heterosexual-familial-masculine subject is the "canonical identity" of the person. Any violation of this norm is understood as "perversion," as "corruption" and hence deserves marginalization or discrimination, even though within this canonical body desire and pleasure are always under interrogation, since, as Watney argues, "familialism lacks any theory of desire beyond the supposed 'needs' of reproduction" (*Practices* 51). This reason explains why gay men and lesbians think or talk about and assert their "sexual identity" far more than heterosexuals, resort more often to activism that is projected from time to time through the gay liberation (or freedom) movement to get sociopolitical status that is identical to that of their heterosexual counterparts. In fact, the gay liberation movement highlighting the "personal" side of lesbians and homosexuals in the US began following the Stonewall riot on June 28, 1969, in which drag queens of Greenwich Village in New York attacked policemen who regularly raided a gay bar called the Stonewall Inn. In the 1970s, homosexuality was decriminalized. The American Psychiatric Association removed homosexuality from its list of classified mental illnesses in 1973. Homosexuality has been recently legalized in the form of monogamous "marriages" in some countries because of pressure from the gay males and females. For example, the same-sex marriages are legal in Belgium, Canada. The Netherlands, South Africa and Spain. Despite this, "homophobia" persists. With the emergence of HIV/AIDS in the 1980s, homosexuality in the US was once again seen as something that was pathological, though it was not officially so. In effect, HIV/AIDS at one level incited homophobia so much so that it caused some categories of panicky gays either to closet themselves away in their rooms or to hide their identities in public. At another level, the disease worked to serve socially as liberation of gay identities from the closet through discourses of resistance to the dominant notion and through activism.

The label GRID was seen as the legalization of the heterosexual canon. Gay men were defined as the victims of their own sexual practices. They were looked upon as those who had HIV/AIDS. For example, in the early years of the epidemic in the US, an anonymous surgeon made a statement, "We used to hate faggots on an emotional basis. Now we have a good reason" (qtd. in Crimp 8). The televangelist Jerry Falwell said, "AIDS is God's judgment of a society that does not live by His rules" (qtd. in Crimp 8). Patrick J. Buchanan, the conservative columnist and speechwriter for the former American President Nixon explained, "The poor homosexuals - they have declared war upon Nature, and now Nature is exacting an awful retribution" (qtd. in Shilts 311). Professor Opendra Narayan of The Johns Hopkins Medical School stated, "These people have sex twenty to thirty times a night [...]. A man comes along and goes from anus to anus and in a single night will act as a mosquito transferring infected cells on his penis. When this is practised for a year, with a man having three thousand sexual intercourses, one can readily understand this massive epidemic that is currently upon us" (qtd. in Bersani 197).

Issues concerning sexual identity that have continually been debated in academic discourses were discussed in the media, among politicians and public health officials following the disease's "gayness" implied in the term GRID. The end-result was that already culturally stigmatized homosexuality itself was feared "as if it were a communicable, lethal disease" (Brandt 155). This notion coupled with the phobic construction of homosexual behaviours (such as fisting, rimming and so on) intensified "homophobia." Cindy Patton in *Inventing AIDS* writes:

> Homophobia is a holograph of fears: fear of a different subculture, fear of forbidden male-male desires, fear of anal penetration. Symbolically, AIDS has collapsed gay sexuality and straight sexual anxiety under the sign of anal sex. Somewhere deep in our representational scheme, the anus is constructed as the quintessential forbidden organ of male-male desire [...]. Strangely enough, [...] the anus is not understood as a sexual organ. [...] The anus's forbidden status [...] combine[s] with the anus's lack of gender reference. Thus, desires centering on the anus cannot infallibly be stabilized to produce 'heterosexuality' and anal sex becomes a key site of (hetero)sexual danger through loss of gender reference.[...] anal sex among heterosexuals must be explained away as a form of birth control, as an uncivilized 'mistake' about where to put 'it,' or as a kinky pleasure engaged in only with 'prostitutes.' (118)

This homophobic gaze of the heterosexuals was marked in the stubborn muteness of the Reagan administration over the epidemic from1981 to 1987 during which nearly 21000 Americans were already dead from the disease, and more than 36000 were diagnosed HIV positive (Shilts 596). The then federal government of the US, scientists, the public health authorities, and the mass media continued to play with American lives affected by HIV/AIDS that was then "projected to claim 365,000 American casualties [...]" (Shilts 618). In those years, it was only gays who started mobilizing resources from among themselves for their treatment, for scientific research on HIV/AIDS, for the management of the disease. Hollywood actor Rock Hudson who was gay and a close friend of the American President Ronald Reagan died of HIV/AIDS in October

1985. Hudson's death "put a human face on the epidemic for many Americans [...]" (Brandt 154).

What infects a celebrity usually affects a nation. With the death of Hudson "AIDS" became a household name in America. The post-Hudson status of HIV/AIDS was significantly different, with the formation of the American Foundation for AIDS Research (AmFAR) funded by contributors like Hudson himself and actress Elizabeth Taylor. However, Hudson's death also aggravated homophobia nationwide with greater force and frequency, thereby utterly stigmatizing the homosexuals. Despite the repeated statements from scientists and epidemiologists that HIV cannot be transmitted through contact, in June 1986 the Justice Department of the US in its ruling authorized employers to bar persons with HIV/AIDS from work, since they were considered "dangerous" to others. This raised a debate on "the rights of the individual to fundamental civil liberties versus the notion of the public good and the role of the state in assuring public welfare"(Brandt 157).

This conflict was seen in the indifference of the Reagan administration (1981-89), the public health officials and researchers at the National Institutes of Health (NIH) to the epidemic. It was also seen in anti-sodomy laws like closure of gay bath houses, in deliberate budget cuts for AIDS research, in plans and proposals to encourage discrimination in employment, housing and the availability of health and life insurance apparently for gays. Many lost jobs, housing and social support. In mid-1983, Edward Grant, the then assistant secretary of health and human services of the federal government declared that HIV/AIDS would be the nation's "number-one" priority. Despite this, because of its close connection with homosexuality, the disease was viewed with suspicion from 1981 to 1986. Practically nothing except the rhetoric prevailed, since, as Allan M. Brandt observes, "Funding for the research and treatment of sexually transmitted diseases has always been suspect in the federal health budget" (162). The proposal to introduce the enzyme-linked immunosorbent assay (the ELISA or popularly known as the "AIDS Test") as a "mandatory" practice for the testing and screening of HIV antibody was aimed at isolating the individuals testing positive. As the then US senator Jesse Helms had put it, "The logical outcome of testing is a quarantine of those infected" (qtd. in Crimp 8). The columnist William F. Buckley wrote, "Everyone detected with AIDS should be tattooed on the upper forearm, to protect common needle users, and on the buttocks to prevent the victimization of other homosexuals" (qtd. in Crimp 8).

This issue got a great deal of adverse publicity in the media, a publicity that then impacted greatly on public perception of the disease. For example, while locating the geography of HIV/AIDS, homosexuals, IV drug users and Haitians were categorized as "city-dwellers." This gave rise to a feeling that HIV/AIDS was a disease of "cities" that traditionally symbolize disease and degeneration. As Gilman notes, "It is the plague of cities after the biblical icon of Sodom and Gomorrah. Righteous Abraham, who dwells in a tent, is contrasted in Genesis with the sinful dwellers in the city [...]. We know where corruption lives, in the city. And purity lives where our fantasy has it that nature (and therefore goodness) dominates: on the farm and in the small town" (266). This geographical perception of the urban as against the rural had also caused differential identities of the HIV-positive people who were seen as the drug-using, homosexual and urban communities. The "country" in HIV/AIDS discourse was privileged as the place of health and safety. In actuality, in the context of industrialization, the "city" is generally seen as a location connected with wealth, permissiveness, development and job opportunities, whereas the country is viewed as a place associated with poverty, restrictiveness, underdevelopment and lack of opportunities. This popular belief is often linked to the epidemic to establish a theory that migrants or drifters are the carriers of HIV. In order to find employment and to get rich quick, people from the rural areas' move to the cities. In the liberal environment of the cities, it is presumed, the poor villagers get involved in multiple activities and relationships, try to internalize citified lifestyle and in doing so acquire HIV/AIDS that is subsequently transmitted to country folk.

Even "lesbians" (female-female desire and sex) were, without any logic, equated with gay men and viewed as a high-risk group for HIV/AIDS. In 1982-83 the American Red Cross postponed accepting gay and lesbian blood donors. In 1987 Sonoma County (California) Red Cross refused to accept the proposal from the lesbians for blood donation drive. However, in actuality, there is the lowest reported incidence of HIV infection among lesbians to date. "Bisexuals" were perceived as invariably homosexual males posturing as heterosexuals and were seen to have acted as "carriers" of HIV. Heterosexuals were considered as the "outside" of the disease's defined limits termed as "risk groups" that obviously included then the stereotyped and stigmatized "non-heterosexuals." When HIV/AIDS was recurrently discovered in categories like IV drug users, hemophiliacs, Haitians and finally heterosexuals, its genesis was ascribed to the sexual practices of homosexuals who were singularly blamed. Only anus was thought to be the breeding ground for HIV. The term "AIDS -victim" used frequently by the press, the public, the government and the medical profession even stood "solely" for homosexuals who, in turn, insisted on being identified or designated as "Person with AIDS (PWA)" or as "people living with AIDS (PLWA)," since the label "victim" has connotations of defeatism, powerlessness, lack of respect, dignity, compassion and understanding.

The term "general population" was a diplomatic euphemism for "heterosexual community," since it did not reveal sexual practices or identities. It, in fact, excluded gays, junkies, IV drug users and lesbians who being the professed non-heterosexuals used the word "heterosexual" in their circles. It was used by the public health officials, politicians and media. Its implication can be understood in the statement of Gary Bauer, President Ronald Reagan's assistant who said in 1985, "It hadn't spread into the general population yet" (qtd. in Grover 23). Bauer made this statement to state the reason behind the "silence" of the President over AIDS that had already spread with staggering speed causing mortality in different parts of America. Thus, the term incorporated hegemonic heterosexuals who were then presumed to be not the "persons with or living with AIDS." As Grover points out, "heterosexuality becomes the mirror of the victimized minority community, besieged from without" (25).

However, the shift in concern over "heterosexual" transmission of HIV/AIDS - a concern associated with the threat that the virus might pass to the majority of people - recognized both penetrative anal and vaginal sex as "routes" of transmission, giving rise to male-to-male, male-to-female and female-to-male categories. These were all clinically, epidemiologically and statistically defined categories, by extension, identities. Following the discovery of large number of HIV-positive people in "heterosexual" denomination, President Reagan for the first time delivered his speech on the disease sometime in mid-1987 and thereby officially recognized HIV/AIDS as a vast problem.

After the entry of "women" into HIV/AIDS, the disease was discussed from different perspectives. Traditionally in patriarchy, as Paula Treichler has pointed out, "disease itself is assigned a female identity" (43). This notion is easily discernible in cases of venereal disease. Ironically, when HIV/AIDS at its initial stage was termed as "gay disease," women were thought to be "inefficient" or "incompetent" transmitters of the disease for biological reasons. After it was established that women are also capable of transmitting the disease, the anxiety of the heterosexual majority about their own potential risk of being infected with HIV/AIDS grew intense. As a result, the term "heterosexual" was substituted by "women" considered not "normal," which included "'prostitutes,' 'drug abusers,' minority and poor women, and women in the Third World" (Treichler 63). The category "prostitutes" was created to keep intact the respectability of all "good" women that included wives, mothers, daughters and sisters. As Grover stresses, "[...] prostitutes are taken as embodiments of infectiousness less for their actual risks and rates of infection than for their symbolic and historical status" (26). Here it may be mentioned that the term "prostitutes" is now replaced by the polite and non-discriminatory phrase "commercial sex workers." The infection of men is often shown as having its source in sexual promiscuity or corruption of women. Arguing this from a feminist position, Treichler writes, "For women, epidemics are rarely benign" (45).

With the increase in heterosexual transmission, sexual practices such as penetrative sex were considered risky. Hence the "risk group" concept was replaced by the non-discriminatory phrase "risk practice." However, the press and the politicians kept emphasizing "risk groups" that functionally concealed, while including, heterosexual men and women and highlighted gay men.

These keywords had a strong adverse hold over the minds of Americans of the 1980s. For example, on recommendation from a special commission of the Reagan administration, as Douglas Crimp in his essay "AIDS: Cultural Analysis/Cultural Activism" notes, laws were passed to forbid lesbians and gay men to adopt children and hence to become potential foster parents. It came at a time when only gay people were willing to parent HIV-positive children. Gay parents were declined guardianship of their natural children "solely on the grounds of sexual orientation." "Gay parenting" and "gay parents" were under severe attack (15). There were other instances also. A thirteen-year old haemophiliac named Ryan White contracted HIV through blood transfusion. He was not allowed to attend the school in Indiana, since angry parents of his schoolmates fearing infection of their children boycotted the school. There was another case in Queens, New York, where the City Board of Education was sued for allowing a seven-year-old child with AIDS to go to school. There was yet another instance. The hous : of the Rays was torched and destroyed when their infected children were allowed to attend the school in Florida in 1987. These children were haemophiliacs and were infected with HIV through blood transfusion. Even now, HIV-positive people all over the world have been targets of violent attacks in certain areas, despite cautions taken by governments and the mass media not to project stigma-centric representations of the disease and not to isolate the affected people from the mainstream. Even though stigma and discrimination have been minimized to a greater extent because of interventions from the governmental and non-governmental help organizations, they are still not allowed to lead a normal life and to contribute meaningfully to the society in certain regions.

Many heroes, as Randy Shilts in his book *And the Band Played On: Politics, People, and the AIDS Epidemic* has shown, had continually fought against the indifferent Ronald Reagan government. In November 1987, AIDS activists heightened campaign for the awareness of the HIV/AIDS crisis. A poster with the words SILENCE=DEATH as logo that was accompanied by a pink triangle being simultaneously the homosexual persecution symbol during the Nazi period and the post-1960 gay liberation emblem appeared on Broadway of New York. The AIDS Coalition to Unleash Power (ACT UP), a nonpartisan HIV/AIDS activist group of diverse but united individuals including heterosexuals in its commitment to direct action to end the epidemic crisis had demonstrated through the slogan "Act Up, Fight

Back, Fight AIDS." It put a neon light symbol entitled "Let the Record Show" that displayed photos, statements and texts evidencing inaction of the Reagan administration and the death toll from HIV/AIDS in the window of New York's New Museum of Contemporary Art. Another group in New York called Testing the Limits videotaped AIDS activism in response to government inaction and produced documentaries that were programmed for viewing at the New Museum along with the window display of the ACT UP.

Gay activists, the ACT UP, clinics, the Centers for Disease Control (CDC), the media and various voluntary service organizations like Shanti Project and Gay Men's Health Crisis pressurized the then American administration to contain HIV/AIDS. As a result, "safe sex," "family," "Just Say No" programmes, ELISA Test for antibodies and health education were chosen belatedly as the preventive and regulatory measures of health policy. Unquestionably, epidemic diseases require prevention and control as long as there is no cure. Microsoft founder Bill Gates and American Presidents like Bill Clinton and George Bush have donated huge amounts of money for the HIV/AIDS prevention and for the rehabilitation of HIV- positive people all over the world. Despite these gestures, HIV positive cases were on the rise in 2008. As reported in the June 3, 2008 edition of the *Times of India*, 33.2 million people were living with HIV worldwide, and around 7,000 people were infected everyday. About 90% of the women got infected with HIV/AIDS by their husbands. This shows that the people's behaviour and attitude concerning sex are unsafe. Even though spread of the disease has now been curbed, it is necessary to revisit and examine critically the above key phrases used for the HIV/AIDS prevention for generation of appropriate awareness in society.

The keyword "safe sex" means avoidance of infected semen in anus or vagina. It focuses on the use of condom that was originally introduced for birth control and family planning. This condom-centric prevention is disapproved by the feminists on the ground that it is centered on the male sexual organ that, as Singer argues, "[...] must be clothed in circulation" (84). Condom foregrounds the safety and protection of the male identity. Singer contends that the term "safe sex" implies that "sex was safe before AIDS [...] as long as it was mostly women who died for and from sex in childbirth, illegal abortions, faulty contraception, rape and murder at the hands of their sexual partners" (67). When Margaret Sanger in the US, for instance, distributed condoms to make sex safer for women dying from bearing too many children or from illegal abortions, she was jailed. This is at one level.

At another level, as Tamsin Wilton has shown, "condom use is feminizing" (34). It threatens "ideologically" the security of the masculine identity. Safe sex mediated through technology causes a barrier between bodies, desires and pleasures, entails both restraint over the man's sexual behaviour and concern for his safety during coition and is thus seen as passivating. "Masculinity" is defined in hetero-patriarchy in terms of the ability to penetrate to effect unmediated penis-in-vagina ejaculation that is emblematized as "real, adult sex" as against non-penetrative, oral and non-genital sex that is labelled as "foreplay" (Wilton 34). This accounts for men's reluctance to use condoms or to engage in non-penetrative sex. The female condom introduced in recent years is viewed as the "empowerment" of women who now do not have to depend on men for protection from infection. Its use ensures full protection for women against sexually transmitted diseases, including HIV/AIDS. It makes women absolutely free from concern about the unsafe sex practices of men on whom now lies the onus to protect themselves by always wearing condom. However, its initial discomfort and difficulty explains its status as bar between bodies, desires and orgasmic pleasures during sex. Consequently, it works to generate unwillingness for sexual practice. This safety guard for women is not also well tolerated by men who occasionally want to experience legal or illegal fatherhood. Particularly women whose only source of livelihood is to have sex with their customers on payment are often threatened with violence and abandonment by men. These ideological interpretations seek to discourage condom use.

For the moral majority, the term "safe sex" promotes promiscuity and destroys family values. For them, instruction for condom use and free distribution of condoms serve only to "condone" indiscriminate sexual practices (anal and vaginal) in certain age groups. For lesbians, the use of "dental latex or dam"as a prophylactic device is ridiculous, since knowledge of woman-to-woman transmission of HIV has not yet been widely accepted and disseminated.

The term "family" as yet another preventive concept in HIV/AIDS discourse is used as "a locus of certainty, of moral and social purity, a zone exempt from conflicts and contagion [...]" (Grover 23). This was evident, for example, in Doolittle's law in 1986. As an HIV prevention measure, the then California State Senator John Doolittle in the legislative session sponsored a bill legalizing blood donors from within families only (and not from any unknown circle). It passed without a single opposition vote. Doolittle's law clearly implied that the family could not be the carrier of HIV. It had also no reference to the families containing gay and lesbian children, parents and IV drug users. Its indirect implication was that those infected with HIV had already been forced to leave the family and were easily identifiable. The law therefore idealistically suggested pristine "purity" contained in the notion of "family."

For the feminists, "family" has only domesticated, reproductive, monogamous, marital, heterosexual and legally recognized paternal values. In this value system, woman's labour as wife, mother, caregiver to man and to her children is always unpaid. In this way, her freedom of body, desire and pleasure is controlled and marginalized by man. Thus, marriage is, as Linda Singer puts it, "the most cost-effective way to maximize the profit potential of women for men, while maintaining a ceiling on the level of male capitalization" (55). The "family" concept has solely reproductive objective. It therefore seeks to ignore the notion of desire and pleasure and to disregard completely the already marginalized "same-sex desire" of gays and lesbians. It, in the process, erases homosexual subjectivity or identity within the systemic power of heterosexuality whose fate "has been and remains indissolubly linked to the fate of patriarchy, capital, and the master race" (Yingling 109). For the live-in partners (of both the same and opposite sexes), marital or family life is bondage. For the mobile and multiple sex partners, family makes no sense, is just a social label that rather serves to hide promiscuity or numerous sexual activenesses.

The phrase "Just Say No" to IV drugs and anonymous sex was a slogan coined by the then US first lady Nancy Reagan. It was considered puritanically moralizing, anti-sexual and impracticable especially in an age of sexual revolution. Its obvious message - abstinence, celibacy, monogamous sexuality - serves to satisfy the dominant ideology of the Moral Majority. This slogan was seen as a repressive mechanism and as encouraging illegal drug use, since the behaviour of IV drug users is impossible to control.

In the post-capitalist commodity culture of the US, these HIV/AIDS prevention strategies were seen as the disciplinary apparatuses to medicalize and regulate "free" sexuality. Despite the criticisms, for the lack of cure of HIV/AIDS, any rational and non-judgmental "prevention" strategy is the one and only option left to make bodies, desire and pleasure come together "safely" in the epidemic period to maintain sexual identities and practices.

The above discussion on HIV/AIDS tropes shows that there is always a slippage between the disease and the representation, between the illness transmission modes and the categorization, between the epidemic and power, between the disease prevention-and-control strategies and the politics of repression. This also shows that disciplinary mechanism subsumed under the disease tropes incites what it seeks to contain. As Linda Singer argues, "[...] disciplines function as enabling forces for inciting and stylizing what they also come to regulate" (74). "Control" seeks always to criminalize behaviour that goes against the norm of the society or State, since it is deployed as power to hold in check certain people who, in turn, choose to resist. Power operates as law. Power-as-law, as Michel Foucault writes, "is always-already present, constituting that very thing which one attempts to counter it with" (*History* 82). This scheme is always at work in all diseases, let alone HIV/AIDS, proliferating in turn endless questions of "identities." HIV/AIDS discourse is evidence of this.

V

"Identity" inherently requires the telling of its "stories" to prove that it exists not in the abstract but in the concrete, in a given space and time. It needs to be remembered for its "perpetuation" through memorializing and narrativizing what it was, has not been, cannot say and cannot be. It is made "meaningful," "recognizable," "communicable" and "recuperative" as an experience in this way and, in the process, is liberated from being a "mere" lackadaisical piece of historical information or document. "Identities" generated by the linguistic and political representations of HIV/AIDS also need the telling of their stories to save them from being pushed into social and cultural information, atrophy, alienation and oblivion. As Yingling points out, "It is only [...] - in the making of artifacts about AIDS - that the disease can become meaningful in a way that allows those affected and infected by it to secure it as an experience and not merely as information. It allows as well an affirmation of identity [...]" (54).

For this reason, it is crucial to have HIV/AIDS narratives, both fictional and nonfictional from everybody including the HIV positive people themselves. Narrativization done differently in oral, written, photographic and audio-visual modes is an act of representation, is required to fulfil the instinctive and inherent need for it in human beings in order to give "sense" to their world of "experience." Through this is affirmed, reinforced and created both an "identity" of the self and a "culture" about the existence of a being. It takes into account both the inside (psychological) and outside (social) of the subject. In other words, it deals with how one sees oneself and is seen by others. In this way, as Madan Sarup points out, "the stories we tell are often reshaped in/for the public sphere. And then, when these narratives are in the public sphere, they shape us" (18). This then raises the question of who tells the story, of what is told in the story and of how the story is told. These questions are the trajectories that constitute the structural and functional dynamics of a narrative. Narrative as a communication is thus a cluster of an addresser (narrator or implied author), an addressee (narrate or implied audience), plot, central event, subplot and so on. Just as identity of a person can be arranged in multiple ways (for example, someone's gender, language, class, race, ethnicity, religion, nation and so on), narrative can also be organized in many ways by its author (for instance, several plots can be created from one story.). Human identity is objectified in narrative that, in turn, is implicated in the expression and production of the subjectivities of individuals. Therefore, narrative and identity are closely interlinked.

Narrative entails storytelling. In storytelling, be it fictional or nonfictional (historical or auto/biographical), is expressed or constituted the "understanding" of the self, whether that of a person or of a community, and "self-understanding is an interpretation; interpretation of the self, in turn, finds in the narrative, among other signs and symbols, a privileged form of mediation [...]"(Ricoeur 114). Thus, through the narrative interpretation of the self is sought the "identity" of the self, an identity that covers entire human life marked as and by indeterminacy or instability of meanings. As Peter Brooks notes, "The question of identity [...] can be thought only in narrative terms, in the effort to tell a whole life, to plot its meaning by going back over it to record its perpetual flight forward, its slippage from the fixity of definition [...]" (33).

The question of HIV positive identity for its appropriate understanding and interpretation, therefore, can be very effectively addressed in HIV/AIDS narratives. In such disease narratives the illness finds voice, is told, heard, read and written from multiple perspectives. Here it can be stated that there has already been a spurt of HIV/AIDS narratives in the West since the late 1980s. These narratives are offshoots of the semiotic, cultural and political projections of HIV/AIDS as the debilitating, stigmatizing and fatal illness in personal life and as the sexual epidemic spreading in collective life due to "deviant" lifestyles and unsafe sexual behaviour and attitude. They depict the self-perceptions of those who are diseased, the representations of those who are not diseased, the resistance to stigma and discrimination and thereby define multiple and mobile identities of the HIV positive people. In the process, they fail to answer appropriately the crucial question of HIV positive identity, even though they contribute to the unprejudiced and non-ideological understanding of the problems of the diseased, thereby inspiring care and love in everybody for the ill. However, they will possibly help arrive empirically at what might be called "the epistemic position of HIV positive identity", a position that this chapter has attempted to explore theoretically, even though mortality from the disease has slowed down now.

This book then seeks to explore the narrativization of HIV/AIDS in America. It proposes to examine the practice and intention of narrating HIV/AIDS. The chapters that follow will attempt to examine selected American HIV/AIDS non-fictional and fictional narratives of the 1980s and 1990s.

2

American HIV/AIDS Nonfiction

In consonance with the framework of the preceding chapter, this one will explore the understandings of "identity" in American HIV/AIDS nonfictional narratives. Nonfiction as a category of literature excludes the nonfactual or the invented. It is expressed in such genres as autobiography, biography, memoir, journal (diary), letter and reporting that need a sketchy review for the purpose of present study.

"Autobiography" is a personal account of one's own life. It is what Laura Marcus calls, "self-life-writing" (294). In it, the first person singular pronoun "I" that both narrativizes and is narrativized is accepted to be alive at the time of giving a continuous account of its own self. The autobiographical "I" is understood to be the knower and the known. Autobiographical impulses and intentions are the offshoots of the autobiographer's attempts to grasp the self, to communicate or explain that self to others, and to define and structure as well the nature of "selfhood" and "identity"all at the same time. These obviously must vary from person to person, since they depend on the way individuals experience their lives in different social, cultural and political settings. They are usually seen as addressing a problem and a solution as well. They engender multiple themes in autobiography, themes that entail multidisciplinary domains of language, truth and knowledge. In this process, autobiography apparently seems to be endlessly unstable and hybrid. However, autobiography at once transcends categorizations and classifications, since "the identity of autobiography is seen as a precondition or guarantor of a remedy for the fractured identity of modernity" (Marcus 7). "Biography" is the another person's account of the life of a person narrativized in proper noun and in third person singular pronoun. However, there is affinity between autobiography and biography. Marcus observes, "Recounting one's own life almost inevitably entails writing the life of an another or others; writing the life of another must surely entail the biographer's identifications with his or her subject, whether these are made explicit or not" (273-74).

"Memoir" is a historical account or biography based on personal knowledge. In other words, it is a written account of events that one has lived through or of the life or character of a person whom one knew. It is also an autobiography or an account of one's memory of certain events or people. However, formally autobiography is "the evocation of a life as a totality, and 'memoirs' [...] offer only an anecdotal depiction of people and events" (Marcus 3). In memoir, memory plays a crucial role. "Journal" or "Diary" is a daily record of events or thoughts, whereas "letter" is a written or printed communication or message addressed to somebody or organization and is usually sent by post, messenger, e-mail or fax. These two are written for personal or official intentions and motivations. They are narrated in first person singular or plural pronoun that is the author or narrator. "Reporting" is the act of stating, narrating, describing, or repeating (especially in the capacity of an eyewitness or hearer) events as facts or as news for the press and for broadcasting and telecasting. Journalism is narrated in proper noun and third person singular or plural pronoun. The pronominal perspectives of these discourses show that the only "I" is the inside, the personal, whereas the others (such as "he," "she," "it" and "they") are the outside, the social or cultural. As has been argued in Chapter-I, the interaction between the "I" and the other pronouns is bound to happen. This suggests collaboration between the autobiographical and the biographical in almost all discourses. This interaction is perhaps the only space or the mediating zone where "identity" of all pronouns exists or is represented and established.

Considering the interactive logic, it can be argued, these nonfictional forms of discourses aiming singularly and assuredly at non-fictive self-revelation through the depiction of life-stories also maintain autobiographical and biographical "agreement" or tie-up and thereby form an indistinguishable suture between the author, the narrator and the narrated self (often called protagonist). Thus, the stories whether true or false always ring true, since they look like autobiographies and biographies that ultimately serve to, as Marcus points out, "structure an uncertain identity into purposive form"(23). American HIV/AIDS nonfiction such as autobiography, biography, memoir, diary and reporting also organizes unspecific identity into certain shape. They are usually non-hierarchical and counter-dominant HIV/AIDS discourses that seek to demonstrate primarily how HIV/AIDS has supplied a site for thorough disclosure and surveillance of privacies, practices and theories of the people, how the disease has mooted the questions of personal, cultural and political identities. In defining the "identity" of the HIV-positive people, they also seek to have the experience of the disease recognized and communicated more meaningfully, to recuperate what has been lost, to save someone else from suffering in the HIV/AIDS epidemic.

In the light of the above, four American HIV/AIDS nonfictional narratives of the 1980s and 1990s are selected for their appropriateness in form and content to develop a contextual and coherent argument in regard to identity-based questions triggered by the HIV/AIDS epidemic in the US. The texts are arranged in order of their "thematic" importance rather than their years of publication for coherence of the argument. The texts examined are *And the Band Played On: Politics, People, and the AIDS Epidemic* by Randy Shilts, *Borrowed Time: An AIDS Memoir* by Paul Monnette, *This Wild Darkness* by Harold Brodkey and *My Own Country: A Doctor's Story* by Abraham Verghese.

Gay journalist Randy Shilts wrote his classic book *And the Band Played On: Politics, People, and the AIDS Epidemic* in 1987. As the first full-time HIV/AIDS reporter in the US, he devoted almost all his time to covering the HIV/ AIDS epidemic during the 1980s in the United States for the *San Francisco Chronicle*. This book is an offshoot of HIV/AIDS news stories that Shilts reported for this newspaper. Shilts clarifies this: "This book is a work of journalism. There has been no fictionalization. For purposes of narrative flow, I reconstruct scenes, recount conversations and occasionally attribute observations to people with such phrases as 'he thought' or 'she felt.' Such references are drawn from either the research interviews I conducted for the book or from research conducted during my years of covering the AIDS epidemic for the *San Francisco Chronicle*"(623).

His narrative of the HIV/AIDS epidemic thus is the true document, the authentic story. However, Douglas Crimp in his essay "How to Have Promiscuity in an Epidemic" considers Shilts's technique of reconstructing different situations through serial episodes as "conventional novelistic fashion" (244). He argues that even though Shilts chronologizes the events ever since the disease appeared and then was inscribed as public or national issue, he poses more like an omniscient narrator than a historian in his attempt to reveal the thoughts, feelings, dreams and nightmares of his characters, of even those who are on the verge of death from HIV/AIDS. Despite his criticism on the fictionalization of fact - a contradiction inherent in Shilts's own clarification given above - Shilts's book apparently makes a convincing case for and hence lays the foundation of the historical account of HIV/AIDS in America during the 1980s. It does so in its "biographical" mode of narrating politics and people in relation to the HIV/AIDS epidemic. Another exonerating feature of the book is its ethical concern. Shilts states his narrative intention, "It is a tale that bears telling, so that it will never happen again, to any people, anywhere" (xxiii). However, these issues have bearing on intricacies and authentication of structures and agencies of identities engendered by HIV/AIDS that finds detailed and vivid expression in this narrative.

The complexities involved in structures and agencies concerning identities that have theoretically been discussed in Chapter-I have been explored here through the key metaphor "band" in the title of the book. The term "band" in the context of the HIV/AIDS epidemic means an organized group of people having a common object. The band obviously included members who expressed indifference, ineptitude and speculation. It simply kept harping on HIV/AIDS without any action-oriented, attitude-change initiative or policy to contain the disease. Till 1988 in regard to the HIV/AIDS prevention, control and research, "in Congress, in the White House, at the National Institutes of Health, and in the media, very little had fundamentally changed. The band still played on" (618). In the context of Silts's observation it is important to note that the United States administration (the Congress and the White House) has the U.S. Department of Health and Human Services (HHS) that runs many health and scientific research agencies, such as the National Institutes of Health (NIH), the Food and Drug Administration (FDA) and the Centers for Disease Control (CDC) that comprise the umbrella name, the U.S. Public Health Service (PHS). Shilts shows that the then federal government of the US, scientists, the public health authorities and the mass media were on top of the band who continued to play with American lives affected by HIV/AIDS that was then "projected to claim 365,000 American casualties [...]" (618).

The then "American government" under conservative Republican President Ronald Reagan was the worst and the cruelest regime in the history of HIV/AIDS. Because of his obstinate heterosexism with pro-family and anti-gay agenda, Reagan was callous and did not care to utter the word "AIDS" for quite some years even after the death of nearly 21000 Americans from the disease, since he believed it to be simply a "gay" disease. The whole Reagan Administration viewed HIV/AIDS as a "budget problem," did not fund any AIDS research by scientific establishments, and deliberately let people die in thousands from the disease without proper care and treatment. Shilts writes, "But [...] saving lives had never been a priority of the Reagan administration. [...] Already, some said that Ronald Reagan would be remembered in history books for one thing beyond all else: He was the man who had let AIDS rage through America, the leader of the government that when challenged to action had placed politics above the health of the American people" (595).

The perception of HIV/AIDS as a homosexual disease initially deterred some American government scientists at the NIH from engaging in research, since the study of the disease, it was feared, would cost them their prestige. However, much later some scientists devoted their attention to the disease and research just for earning nation-wide or global recognition, name and fame for themselves. Robert Gallo, for instance, was interested more in winning the Nobel prize for his unjustified claim as the "sole" discoverer of the AIDS virus than in collaborating with international (mainly European) AIDS research efforts undertaken much earlier by the French scientist Luc Montagnier who was the first discoverer of HIV. By the time the dispute between Montagnier and Gallo was resolved in the form of naming them both as the "co-discoverers" of HIV, the core issue of fighting against the disease itself was brushed aside and, as a result, people suffered and died.

The "careful" case-control studies of the CDC, studies that were actually devised with the best of intentions to control the epidemic created and, in effect, victimized HIV/AIDS categories such as homosexuals, hemophiliacs, heroin addicts, Haitians and prostitutes from time to time. Homosexuals were made the number-one target of victimization. Political and public interpretations of the CDC data and categories spawned God's judgement, Nature's retribution and quarantine theories targeting gays from the religious fundamentalist Jerry Falwell with his Moral Majority, right-wing columnist Patrick Buchanan and the conservative U.S. senator Jessie Helms respectively. The "conservatives" of these varieties who used extensively moralizing terms to denigrate gays and to inflame homophobia also constituted the members of the band that played on in the HIV/AIDS epidemic. Their pronouncements led to the rise of brutal assaults on gays, of discrimination in jobs and in other social and civic privileges and of the denial of health insurance for gays.

Public health authorities being guided by the political leaders saw the disease as a political problem and "refused to take the tough measures necessary to curb the epidemic's spread [...]" (xxii). Basing its findings on five transfusion cases in December, 1982, the Morbidity and Mortality Weekly Report (MMWR), the CDC's weekly newsletter publicly announced for the first time that AIDS "'may be caused by an infectious agent transmitted sexually or through exposure to blood or blood products'"(207). Blood bankers were angry. Shilts writes, "In spite of that, Dr. Joseph Bove, who headed the FDA's blood advisory committee and served as an officer of the American Association of Blood Banks, went on network television to say flatly that there still was no evidence that transfusions spread AIDS. Privately some blood bankers thought the CDC was overstating the possibility of transfusion AIDS to get publicity and, therefore, more funding. [...] Some blood bankers, including some officials of the FDA, remained unconvinced that AIDS even existed" (207).

However, in January 1983 the CDC was bent on controlling the threat HIV posed to the nation's blood supply in two ways. First was through keeping people at high risk from donating blood. Second was through hepatitis B core antibody testing. Hepatitis B core antibodies were abundantly found in the blood of people in the AIDS risk groups (gay men, intravenous drug users and hemophiliacs) who at some point in their lives had been infected with the hepatitis B virus. This simply meant screening of blood for hepatitis B as a surrogate marker for HIV. This second option was considered unfeasible, since the cost of the testing was prohibitively high even for the non-profit blood-bank industry the American Red Cross. The for-profit blood-products (such as Factor VIII) manufacturers were not in favour of the second option. The first option to screen blood donors and to exclude all people in high-risk groups, including gays was firmly opposed by gay rights organizations on grounds of civil rights questions, since donor screening would fuel total stigmatization leading to elimination of all gay men from the donor pool. Shilts writes, "'Direct or indirect questions about a donor's sexual preference are inappropriate,' the statement said. Dr. Roger Enlow, a New York City gay physician and a leader of the American Association of Physicians for Human rights, heralded the policy. 'We've preserved not just gay rights,' he said, 'but the human right to privacy and individual choice'" (224). Frank Kameny, the veteran gay politician remarked, "[...] he would 'advise fellow gays to lie' if the local blood bank officials proceeded with screening"

(238). Thus, gays called for the option of hepatitis B core antibody testing. This stalemate continued and served only to increase infection with and death from HIV/AIDS. By mid-1987, as Shilts writes, "An estimated 12,000 Americans were infected from transfusions largely administered after the CDC had futilely begged the blood industry for action to prevent spread of the disease" (599).

The presumed gayness of HIV/AIDS prevented the mass media in America from discussing all aspects of the disease. American newspapers and televisions occasionally chose to highlight the rightist views. They largely ignored covering stories about the disease until the HIV/AIDS casualties included heterosexuals, Hollywood celebrity Rock Hudson who was gay as well as a friend of President Reagan, and the death toll was too high to ignore. As Shilts puts it, "Without the media to fulfil its role as public guardian, everyone else was left to deal – and not deal – with AIDS as they saw fit"(xxiii).

Shilts himself being openly gay does not spare even gay community and its leaders from being the part of the band. Gay community leaders considered HIV/AIDS public relations problems, "played politics with the disease, putting political dogma ahead of the preservation of human life" (xxii). This needs to be understood through a brief history of the gay liberation movement in the US. Following the Stonewall riot on June 28, 1969, in which drag queens of Greenwich Village in New York attacked policemen who regularly raided a gay bar called the Stonewall Inn, the gay liberation movement highlighting the "personal" side of lesbians and homosexuals in the US began. The gay liberation movement of the 1970s caused the movement of a very large number of gays to San Francisco, gay activism and commercialization of gay sex through institutions like gay bath houses and sex clubs that were usually owned by gay political leaders, were serving to support financially disadvantaged gay groups. Gay freedom and identity were explored through gay sexual revolution. Gay sex acts such as "rimming" were popularized through literature. Shilts observes, "Promiscuity, however, was central to the raucous gay movement of the 1970s, [...]" (19). He also writes, "[...] sex was part and parcel of political liberation" (19). However, the movement succeeded, as Shilts shows, in victimizing itself. Shilts reports, "[...] the bathhouses were a horrible breeding ground for disease. People who went to bathhouses simply were more likely to be infected with a disease - and infect others - than a typical homosexual on the street "(19). A Seattle study showed that by absorbing faeces of the sexual partners from the bathhouses, gay men suffered from shigellosis. According to a Denver study, many had picked up syphilis or gonorrhea from the tubs. These studies were made before HIV/AIDS was discovered. The early 1982 CDC case control study of HIV/AIDS that was then known as gay-related immune deficiency (GRID) revealed that the disease was sexually transmitted, a product of "the fast-lane life-style" of homosexuals, who had frequented gay bath houses, had uncountable sexual partners, had "as many as 20,000 sexual contacts"(132).

Deducing from this, "promiscuity" was presumed to be the source of infection. However, the word was "quickly denounced by gay leaders as 'judgmental'" (258). The advice for safe sex, condom use and avoidance of any exchange of bodily fluids was viewed as the "anti-sexual" and "panic-prone" gestures, as attack on "precious and hard-won" way of gay life and as expression of "internalized homophobia" by gay leaders who wanted gay men to be projected as "sex fiends" in need of their bathhouses. Konstantin Berlandt, the then co-chair of the gay parade board of directors and a columnist for the *Bay Area Reporter* said in mid-1983, "'I didn't become a homosexual so I could use condoms,' [...]. 'Of course, we're concerned about spreading a disease. But what should we do? Take our bodily fluids and put them in barrels [...]?'" (317). He also wrote in late 1983, "'Advice on safe sex, while perhaps well meaning, is actually collaboration with the death regime that delights in blaming ourselves and would pin the blame on us. The myth of 'safe sex' fosters the finger pointing when anyone of us does come down with a disease: 'You see, we told you so. We brought it on ourselves'"' (378). He also spiritualized rimming that was then considered to be the highly risky transmission route for HIV/AIDS, "'I love to rim. To some people, a tongue up the asshole can be relaxing, mesmerizing, even spiritually uplifting'" (378). Shilts adds in his report, "Berlandt maintained it was society's responsibility to find the medical technology to prevent all sexually transmitted diseases, rather than the gay community's responsibility to keep sexuality in line with what medical technology could cure. As for safe sex, he wrote, 'I don't mean we can't make such changes if absolutely necessary, but why must we?'"(378).

A profit-seeking San Mateo doctor assured that he could cure the disease through megadoses of vitamin C. Gay psychologists ruled out sexual transmission of the disease and maintained that "AIDS victims all had suffered an 'emotional emergency' as children that made them feel abandoned. The abandonment now was being played out with AIDS, [...] meaning that change in psychological posture toward the world could be the best prevention against the disease" (378). Suggestions for bathhouse closure and display of safe-sex postures at bathhouses were opposed, since, it was feared, it would cost the gay community their socioeconomic viability. One of the owners of the largest bathhouses reasoned with Drs. Don Abrams and Paul Volberding at San Francisco General Hospital in early 1984, "'We're both in it for the same thing,' [...]. 'Money. We make money at one end when they come to the baths. You make money from them on the other end when they come here'" (422). Embroiled in the controversial issues of civil liberties of gays and of moneymaking attitude of bathhouse owners, all safe sex measures were deferred for several years till 1987, when all bathhouses were closed. In those years of bathhouse controversy, people died and continued to be infected with HIV/AIDS.

The so-called foreign origin theories of HIV/AIDS also could be connected to the band. In their search for sources of the disease, some people speculated about many possibilities and started engaging in accusation. They were doctors, scientists, epidemiologists and perhaps, among others, journalist Randy Shilts himself who saw the origin of HIV/AIDS in some place outisde America. This can be ascertained in the very systematization of stories in Shilts's book itself. The book begins with the story of throngs, including "sailors" and people from "all over the world" in America's 200th birthday celebration on July 4, 1976 in New York. This event is then "immediately" followed by the story of a forty-seven-year-old Danish lesbian doctor Margrethe Rask. There is then the story of a French-Canadian airline steward Gaetan Dugas who was called "patient zero" by the CDC. The book ends with the story of the "'slim'" (621) or HIV/AIDS-infected son of a Ugandan soldier Charles Lwanga. The memories of America's bicentennial birthday celebration that was attended by sailors from fifty-five nations and by people from all over the world were retrieved in mid-1982 to connect them to the onset of HIV/AIDS in America. As Shilts writes, "Nothing happened before 1976, but people had started getting sick in 1978 and 1979. It was clear from the other links in the cluster study that the disease could lie dormant for a long time. People were spreading it all over in 1977 and 1978, which accounted for so many cases spontaneously appearing in so many different regions of the country"(142). The implication was that the disease had been transmitted from non-Americans gathered at the Manhattan celebration. Who were these non-Americans?

Shilts cleverly answers the implied question in the next story of Dr. Grethe Rask, who was from Denmark and was then in charge of a hospital in Zaire in Central Africa. She had worked for four years with Belgian nuns and with "what she could beg and borrow. This was Central Africa, after all, and even a favored clinic would never have such basics as sterile rubber gloves or disposable needles. You just used needles again and again until they wore out; once gloves had worn through, you risked dipping your hands in your patient's blood because that was what needed to be done" (4). Dr. Rask was a lesbian who contracted a disease associated with fatigue, weight-loss, diarrhoea and swollen lymph glands. She died in 1977. The disease was much later diagnosed as HIV/AIDS. Her death indicated African origin of AIDS. The Central Africa was believed to have regularly begotten new diseases. Shilts writes, "The battle between humans and disease was nowhere more bitterly fought than here in the fetid equatorial climate, where heat and humidity fuel the generation of new life forms. One historian has suggested that humans, who first evolved in Africa eons ago, migrated north to Asia and Europe simply to get to climates that were less hospitable to the deadly microbes the tropics so efficiently bred"(5).

In seeking to find out the non-American vectors of HIV/AIDS in America, Shilts writes the story of Gaetan Dugas, a French-Canadian airline steward who was one of the first North-Americans diagnosed with AIDS. Gaetan was a Canadian, a French-speaking Quebecois. He acquired skill in English only to meet the bilingual job requirement for flight attendant in Air Canada. He loved to travel. He had the passes that allowed him to fly all over the world for virtually nothing. He obsessively loved to announce always to his friends and to himself, "'I am the prettiest one'" (21). Despite his narcissistic mindset, he had charmed any male model he used to come across into buggery. Even though he had been adopted and brought up by French-Canadian working class parents in Quebec City, "[...] he had found his own niche in the royalty of gay beauty, as a star of the homosexual jet set" (196). Ever since he developed purple spots that were medically proved as Kaposi's sarcoma in June 1980, his friends and sex mates had frequently asked him about those spots. To avoid embarrassment he shaved his head in order that he would not be easily recognized. To go unidentified during his sexual practices, he kept to cubicles of bathhouses where the lights were dim enough. He adopted this strategy as he traveled between San Francisco, Los Angeles, Vancouver, Toronto and New York. In 1981 the CDC discovered that Gaetan had "250 sexual contacts a year. He'd been involved in gay life for about ten years and easily had had 2,500 sexual partners"(83). In April 1982 the CDC called Gaetan Dugas "Patient Zero" for his statistically proven efficiency to be "zero" in respect of his being both the fountainhead and the prime agency of infection with and spread of HIV/AIDS in America. Doctors statistically concluded that as of April 12, 1982 at least 40 of the first 248 gay men diagnosed with HIV/AIDS in ten cities in the United States had had sex with either Gaetan or men sexually linked to Gaetan. Advised by doctors to stop going to bathhouse to restrict the spread of HIV/AIDS, Gaetan used to argue, "'I've got it,' [...]. 'They can get it too'" (200).

Gaetan's retaliatory logic of giving HIV/AIDS right back to others on grounds of the disease being given to him by somebody could not be held in check despite much persuasion from his best friend from Toronto to give up sex. Shilts writes, "Asking Gaetan to give up sex, [...] would be like asking Bruce Springsteen to give up the guitar. Sex wasn't just sex to Gaetan; sex was who Gaetan was - it was the basis of his identity" (251). Just to infect others with HIV, he intentionally used to have sex. After having sex with willing partners, he would show his Kaposi's sarcoma lesions and say: "'I've got gay cancer,' [...]. 'I'm going to die and so are you'" (165). In addition, questioning the spread of the disease through sex Gaetan argued before the audience, "'[...]. How can people say this can be passed along when they don't even know what causes it?'"(247). After being threatened by a group of gay men in Castro Street (San Francisco) for his bathhouse escapades and for so purposely spreading the disease, Gaetan moved back to Vancouver in Canada. He had survived his fourth bout with pneumocystis and at last died of kidney-failure at the age of 31 in Quebec City of Canada in March 1984. Shilts writes:

> Whether Gaetan Dugas actually was the person who brought AIDS to North America remains a question of debate and is ultimately unanswerable. The fact that the first cases in both New York City and Los Angeles could be linked to Gaetan, who himself was one of the first half-dozen or so patients on the continent, gives weight to that theory. Gaetan traveled frequently to France, the western nation where the disease was most widespread before 1980. In any event, there's no doubt that Gaetan played a key role in spreading the new virus from one end of the United States to the other. The bathhouse controversy, peaking so dramatically in San Francisco on the morning of his death, was also linked directly to Gaetan's own exploits in those sex palaces [...]. At one time, Gaetan had been what every man wanted from gay life; by the time he died, he had become what every man feared. (439)

Shilts's search for the origin of HIV/AIDS in an "alien" Canadian citizen named Gaetan Dugas who in turn was infected with the disease in France reiterates the non-Americanness of the disease, a non-Americanness that is once again stressed in the last heterosexual story of the book. This mid-1987 story is about the second son of Charles Lwanga who was serving in the Ugandan army. Lwanga's son and grandchild as well as another couple were suffering from HIV/AIDS known there as "slim disease." Lwanga "knows only that the United States is a country of immense wealth, and that the medicine that will save his country and his son will probably come from there [...] and he asks, 'When will it come? When will there be the cure?'"(621). This story establishes the African origin of the disease. Elsewhere Shilts writes, "Although evidence of heterosexual AIDS transmission could be dated back to the first epidemiological studies by the Centers for Disease Control in the summer of 1981, it was not until early 1985 that the straight links of the disease garnered much attention. The most disconcerting stories came from Central Africa, where AIDS was simply called 'the horror sex disease'. [...] Ugandans had dubbed AIDS 'slim disease' because of the wasting away that marked the virulent parasitic diseases" (510). Shilts, by subscribing to the foreign origin theory of HIV/AIDS, is of course guilty of deliberately constructing an opposition between America as a rich (and therefore healthy) nation and Africa as a poor (and therefore diseased) continent. He is also marginalizing the status of other nations by privileging the notion of cultural and economic imperialism of the US. For him, HIV/AIDS cannot happen in America. It can only come to America through non-American carriers.

Thus, the metaphor "band" brings into its fold the American government with its political leaders, the scientists, the conservatives, the public health authorities, the mass media, gay community with its leaders and the foreign origin theorists. It has been both structure and agency in the construction of the HIV/AIDS epidemic and of HIV-positive identities. However, Shilts's portrait of gay sexuality and life-style has been viewed as foregrounding homosexuality rather than the American government as the cause of the spread of HIV/AIDS. As, in a review of *And the Band Played On* Michael Fumento remarks, "[...] most historians, with the help of Shilts's book, will conclude that, although many share the blame for the AIDS epidemic, those primarily responsible were its prime victims, the homosexuals themselves." Particularly, the depiction of "Patient Zero" as someone potentially vicious has been seen as the projection of Shilts's own subconscious homophobia despite his gay orientation. By scapegoating Gaetan, as Douglas Crimp in his essay "How to Have Promiscuity in an Epidemic" argues, "Shilts unconsciously identifies with all those who would rather see gay men die than allow homosexuality to invade their consciousness"(244).

Of course, these ways of reading the message of Shilts's book, it may be argued, are the product of gay historical compulsion and necessity. After all, those were the HIV/AIDS-associated years that were juxtaposed with the period of the gay's revolutionary emergence from the closet for the cultural recognition and acceptance of gay identity. Obviously, the gay press had been one of most vital sources of information on all aspects of HIV/AIDS since the commencement of the epidemic. Gaetan Dugas pictured by gay journalist Shilts was therefore accepted as true and reported as such for heterosexual sensation by the "general" news media. This served to inflame and disseminate homophobia and escalated further pathologization and stigmatization of gay identity. At this level, the book was regarded as simply seeking to legitimize the notion of voracious sexuality, murderous irresponsibility of the homosexuals and thereby tried to justify the genocidal gesture of the then Reagan Administration and the denial of gay identity. For this reason, despite the book's status as a bestseller and a nominee for the 1987 National Book Critics Circle Award for Best nonfiction, it was considered disastrous among gays, AIDS activists, people with AIDS and people involved in the struggle against AIDS. Calling the book a "thriller narrative," Douglas Crimp ruthlessly attacks it: "His book contributes nothing to understanding and changing it" ("How to Have" 246).

As a journalist, Shilts has documented the highly sensitive HIV/AIDS story as he has seen and heard it. In his account he has also the stories of a number of scientists, doctors, nurses, public health officials, HIV/AIDS patients and most importantly gay leaders who were "heroes." These heroes risked everything, braved all vilification, fought against the "created" mainstream and community conventions of thrusting rejection, fear and isolation upon the sufferers and were the crusaders of the epidemic with the intention "to make people understand and to make people care" (xxiii). In fact, the first breakthroughs in HIV/AIDS research were made possible owing to funds that gays lobbied for and actually raised among themselves. These gays strongly argued for a sane response to the epidemic from their own community. This was demonstrated, for example, by gay leaders like Bill Kraus, Cleve Jones and Ron Huberman in their letter to The *Bay Area Reporter*: "'Unsafe sex is – quite literally- killing us [...]. Unsafe sex with a number of partners [...] at bathhouses and sex clubs is particularly dangerous [...]. If the gay movement means anything, it means learning self-respect and respect for another. When a terrible disease means that we purchase our sexual freedom at the price of thousands of our lives, self-respect dictates it is time to stop until it once again is safe [...]'" (260). To be self-critical is to be rationally, ethically alert to dangers and not to be against community-centric interest or agenda. In the 21st century, the spirit of this letter is shared globally for the epidemic prevention, since "unsafe" promiscuity has no gender, sexual, communal and national affiliations and is the site of HIV/AIDS. Shilts as a journalist knows his "role as public guardian" (xxiii). The prevention of communal catastrophe requires immediate effective intervention that at times goes against the communal will, since the question of survival precedes everything else. Certainly, Shilts has an apocalyptic vision of the gay world following the HIV/AIDS epidemic and, through the book, makes a case for seamless and healthy growth and continuity of gay identity.

Shilts's history of HIV/AIDS in America is followed by Paul Monette's *Borrowed Time: An AIDS Memoir* (1988) that became yet another bestseller and a nominee for the 1988 National Book Critics Circle Award for best biography. Monette's book is an HIV/AIDS biography. It is written under the acute feeling of Monette's own infection with HIV/AIDS. At the same time, it is also written on the death of his gay lover Roger Horwitz from HIV/AIDS on October 22, 1986. Roger lived for nineteen months and ten days after the diagnosis was mde. In the 1980s, as Shilts's book discussed above has shown, HIV/AIDS known then as "gay disease" affected many and was accompanied by a mounting death toll primarily because of Reagan's indifference. Monette in his book also endorses this as he writes, "Reagan would be remembered, [...] for just one thing, that he presided over the denial of the calamity" (170). On recommendation from a special commission of the Reagan administration, as Douglas Crimp in his essay "AIDS: Cultural Analysis/ Cultural Activism" notes, laws were passed to prevent lesbians and gay men from adopting children. It came at a time when only gay people were willing to parent HIV-positive children. Gay parents were declined guardianship of "their natural children solely on the grounds of sexual orientation" (15). Many heroes, as Shilts's book has shown, had continually fought against the indifferent American government. In November 1987, activists heightened campaign for the awareness of the HIV/AIDS crisis. A poster with the words SILENCE=DEATH as logo appeared on Broadway of

New York. The AIDS Coalition to Unleash Power (ACT UP), a nonpartisan HIV/AIDS activist group of diverse but united individuals including heterosexuals had demonstrated through the slogan "Act Up, Fight Back, Fight AIDS." Another group in New York called Testing the Limits videotaped AIDS activism in response to government inaction and produced documentaries that were programmed for viewing at New York's New Museum of Contemporary Art.

All the apathy and activism preceded and followed 1988, significantly the year of publication of Monette's book. The spirit of the period had remained untold in "writerly" mode by "the diseased" themselves. Against this backdrop, Monette's book breaks new ground in its effort to combine contemporary gay history's spirit of resistance to hold gay identity high with personal experience in relation to HIV/AIDS. For example, it records:

> It was said that everyone appointed by the Reagan administration in a major public health capacity was either a Mormon or a fundamentalist. The chief spokesman for the administration now was the overripe and venomous Patrick Buchanan, one of whose major qualifications for the job was his widely quoted remark that nature was finally exacting her price on homosexuals for having spilled their seed and her. The right-wing firebrands are obsessed with sodomy, always forgetting that half of the gay world is women. This deterministic smugness, whereby we were only getting what we deserved, was so widespread in the upper chambers of the government that the AIDS issue probably never darkened the threshold of the Oval Office. Not to mention the fundamentalists: Though the press would not report anything about the antivirals and wouldn't assess the scope of the death of a

> gay generation, they reported with loving detail every ranting speech of the Falwell-Schlaflys and their money-changing brethren. "God's punishment" was the major level of public debate in 1985: hate, it appeared, was the only public health tool available. (166)

This experience of loathing for homosexuals is sutured on to the deeply personal gay love being invaded by HIV/AIDS. Monette's book transmutes the cultural construction of gay morbidity and mortality into something spiritually salubrious and immortal through the poignantly lyrical love story of Paul and Roger. This is suggested in Monette's choice of the book's title "Borrowed Time," taken from the words of deceased Roger, "We're living on borrowed time, aren't we?" (285). Thus, the title along with the book serving fittingly as a sort of memorial or epitaph stretches Roger, by connotative extension or analogy, HIV-positive gay identity, unexpectedly into protracted deathlessness. This unexpected extension of Roger's life owes its origin to Dr. Denis Cope, who had struggled to save Monette's AIDS-afflicted lover Roger for nineteen months. It was Cope who had inspired Monette to write a biography of Roger to overcome his loneliness and helplessness. When Roger was on the verge of death Paul was nervous, "'What am I going to do without him?' I asked in a hollow voice, and Cope replied immediately, with great force and conviction. 'Write about him, Paul', he said. 'That's what you have to do'" (341). Cope's suggestion is transformed into Monette's resolution immediately following Roger's death. This is suggested in the last sentence of the book, "Putting off as long as I could the desolate waking to life alone - this calamity that is all mine, that will not end till I do"(342). Monette's gratefulness for this piece of advice is shown through his dedication of the book to Denis Cope.

However, Monette's resolution is interrupted by his

own sense of himself being HIV positive when he begins the book with a total sense of gloom and resignation, "I don't know if I will live to finish this. [...] All I know is this: The virus ticks in me. And it doesn't care a whit about our categories - when is full-blown, what's AIDS-related, what is just sick and tired? No one has solved the puzzle of its timing. [...] I used up all my optimism keeping my friend alive. Now that he's gone, the cup of my own health is neither half full nor half empty. Just half" (1-2). Monette's desperate acceptance of the inevitabe effects of HIV/AIDS is confronted by his authorial anxiety about "endings" and "closures." As an HIV/AIDS-biographer he was sure of his own death at any moment in course of his writing, "Equally difficult, of course, is knowing where to start. The world around me is defined now by its endings and its closures - the date on the grave that follows the hyphen" (2). The pathetic helplessness criss-crossing the tragical death of his beloved coupled with the caring doctor's advice coincides with the gay cultural compulsion to liberate gay identity enmeshed then in the escalation of conspiracy, homicide and annihilation theories on the pretext of preventing HIV/AIDS. Monette's narrative thus is written "purely" from gay male perspective with strong historical sense. It is also a way of eternally celebrating gay love.

The gay love is not just between Roger and Paul. The gay lovers who had been living together for six years were not just Roger and Paul. Rather "we were a hyphenate, Roger-and-Paul, such a unified field [...]" (54). The hyphenated gay love, as it proceeds in the narrative, transcends time and space, becomes universal. Monette makes a strong case for developing a "naturally" given or "always-already" notion of gay sexual identity. This is evident when he writes:

> We met on the eve of Labor Day in 1974, at a dinner party [...] just two days before Roger was to start work as an attorney at a stately firm in

> Boston. He was thirty-two; I was twenty-eight [...] and I for one was in love before the night was done. I suppose we'd been waiting for each other all our lives. The business of coming out had been difficult for both of us, partly because of the closet nature of all relations in a Puritan town like Boston, partly because we were both so sure of what we wanted and it kept not coming to life.
>
> [...]
>
> For [...] when we met, everything I'd brooded over from the ancient Greeks to Whitman [...] all ceased to be literary. My life was a sort of amnesia till then, longing for something that couldn't be true until I'd found the rest of me. Is that feeling so different in straight people? Or is it that gay people have to keep it secret and so grow divided, with a bachelor's face to the world and a pang like dying inside? (10-11)

The phrase "from ancient Greeks to Whitman" stands for homosexual orientation of great Greek and American writers that Monette was familiar with through his reading of history and literature. However, Monette raises unanswerable questions about gay and straight identities, and, through this gay love story, persuades predominantly heterosexual society into accepting homosexual identity as a natural thing. This may be read in the heterosexual paradigm as the authorial "politics" of persuasion by language loaded with emotion. However, memoir has no strategy, only demands the representation of "truth" of feeling for the deceased from the survivor, even though HIV/AIDS in its social and cultural interpretation also provides an opportune context for Monette's writing. Elsewhere Monette raises the problem of articulating his understanding of Roger, "How do I speak of the person who was my life's best reason?"(9). This rhetorical question would, at least, for a moment, produce the willing suspension of anti-homosexual notions, even though it is preceded by the candid description of the sexuality of Roger and Paul:

> Roger especially didn't march to the different drum of *so many men,* [...]. In ten years he had perhaps half a dozen contacts outside the main frame of our relationship, mostly when he was out of town on business. He was comfortable with relative monogamy, even at a time when certain quarters of the gay world found the whole idea trivial and bourgeois. I realize that in the world of the heterosexual there is a generalized lip service paid to exclusive monogamy, a notion most vividly honored in the breach. [...] it was difficult enough for us to fashion a sexual ethics just for us. In any case, I was the one in the relationship who suffered from lost time. I was the one who would go after a sexual encounter as if it were an ice cream cone- casual, quick, good bye. (5)

Of course, Monette is critical of the notion of "monogamy" as sexual ethics, since he always hesitated "over the marriage word" (24). Nevertheless, he gives an insightful analysis of their character. By nature Roger is unpretentious and patient, whereas Paul is mercurial and frantic. As Monette puts it, "I am the weather, Roger is the climate, and they are not always the same" (65). Despite attitudinal incompatibility, they can cohabit with great intensity, love and care. This is reflected continuously in the entire period of their relationship as live-in lovers. This was there during their initial two years in the puritan locality of Paul's parental hometown Boston where their homosexual love went unsuspected and unrevealed. This did also prolong in the later period from 1977 when they moved to California owning an apartment house in Los Angeles (LA) with Roger's half-brother Sheldon who was "the most important [...] gay man in California politics"(53).

Sheldon's mother, who was dead, was the first wife of his father Al. His stepmother Bernice and Al were Roger's parents who lived in Chicago and, without their knowledge, were looked upon by Paul as "my in-laws" (51). This marital feeling just happened despite the fact that he did not marry Roger. It can be seen as a sort of plea to revive and legalize ancient "gay marriages" (24). It is perhaps aimed for posterity to do away with the notion that "Everyone gay starts out in the closet, of course" (320). The closet notion of gayhood had gradually been disappearing following the gay liberation movement of the 1970s. It has now been completely eroded by HIV/AIDS that necessitates the surveillance of the most private and intimate practices. This was the reason why Roger's diagnosis of HIV/AIDS gave opportunities for the lovers "to live on the moon" (2). However, as the results of broncoscopy showed evidence of pneumocystis carinii pneumonia (PCP) in the lungs of Roger, Monette reacted, "I ran round the bed and clutched Roger's hand, 'We'll fight it, darling, we'll beat it, I promise. I won't let you die.' The sentiments merged as they tumbled out. This is the liturgy of bonding. Mostly we clung together, as if time still had the decency to stop when we were entwined. After all, the whole world was right here in this room. I don't think Roger said anything then. Neither of us cried. It begins in a country beyond tears. Once you have your arms around your friend with his terrible news, your eyes are too shut to cry" (77).

Roger was also equally concerned about Paul's health. He asked the doctor "What about Paul?"(80). As for Paul, what had happened to Roger should also happen to Paul: "if Roger died then I died" (84). This was the logic of their romance. Unable to bear the separation with Roger who was then in hospital for weeks under his constant bedside care and the doctor's supervision, Monette had cried, contemplated suicide to get rid of pain and bitter despair. He writes, "When you are gay and alone and want to be a poet, suicide crosses your mind [...]" (93-94). However, the need to look after the bedridden Roger deterred him from dwelling on the "easiness of death" (93). After hospitalization, Roger temporarily recovered from AIDS-related diseases and came home. Paul and Roger "made love again [...]" (124). This is apparently a dangerous love, since it is a conscious act of exposing oneself to HIV/AIDS. However, this was symbolic of Monette's defiance of the disease that had subjected gay love to homophobia and stigma:

> Seven years into the calamity, too many gay men have lost the will to love. The enemies of our people – fundamentalists of every stripe, totalitarians left and right—have all been allowed the full range of their twitching bigotry. [...] too many of us have internalized their self-hatred as shame. That the flesh and the spirit are one in love is none of the business of the celibate men of God, especially those who believe they rule the province of love. But the mission of the homophobe is more pernicious even than his morality. He wants every one of us to be all alone, never to find the beloved friend.
>
> [...] two men in love can't rejoice out loud – joy of the very thing everyone burns for - [...]. I try to remember that we fight as a ragged people to outlast the calamity so that others can sleep as safe as my friend and I, like a raft in the tempest. (124-25)

Ironically, at the pre-diagnostic stage Roger was showing symptoms such as flu, amoebiasis, weight loss, cold and cough that were called *"Pre-AIDS"* (31). It had then filled Monette with a sense of guilt: "None of this would be happening if I'd never had sex with strangers. I suppose

I felt there was something innately shameful about dying of a venereal disease" (32). At that stage also Monette had "a perfect frenzy of prophylaxis, almost a phobia" (45). For example, his guest room mattress, which was used for a brief period by his Uruguayan friend Cesar Albini who had full-blown AIDS, was cleaned with ammonia by Paul: "Scared shitless too, because what if everyone was wrong about the virus after all? Maybe it could cling to a pillow slip where a fevered head tossed restless. And if the sweat soaked through the pillow, did you have to throw that out as well?"(45). Only at a much later stage Monette's blood test results had confirmed his "exposure to the AIDS virus" (149).

Roger's diagnosis was not initially disclosed to his parents who might not be able to bear the shock. Nor was it told to anyone, since public disclosure would cost Roger his job as a lawyer in the LA firm, would even deter clients from coming to him for legal advice. "AIDS was that extreme a stigma" (79).

In fact stigma manifests itself in panic, discrimination and denial. Even the medical establishment is not free from this. Monette narrates his own experience with his physician to whom he broke the news that Roger had PCP:

> He shrugged his shoulders with a cavalier unconcern I can only attribute to his certainty that he was safe himself. I've seen that straight man's shrug a hundred times. "Burn the blankets," he replied facetiously, [...].
>
> I felt as if I'd just been run over by a truck, [...]. Is this how a Jew feels when he hears 'holocaust' appropriated to some other calamity?
>
> "You live alone, you die alone," my doctor said sententiously, [...].
>
> Not *us*, I thought, as the rage began to build like a boiling tsunami. My determination to be with

> Rog every minute I could, whatever happened, took stubborn form in the doctor's office. White-hot rage is the only thing that keeps you going sometimes. (85)

Monette records yet another experience with the dental hygienist who reacted to his announcement that he had been exposed to the AIDS virus: "She backed away in abject horror and ran from the room. There was a spate of frantic whispering in the hall, and then the receptionist came in and asked me to move to the main examining room. After a minute Dr. Kurtzman himself came in, obviously shaken but rigorously professional. He expressed genuine sympathy [...], then began the process, awkward for him as much as me, of donning gloves and mask" (113 -14).

This panic situation was also experienced at the University of California in Los Angeles (UCLA) where wearing of masks by dentists was made obligatory. Many AIDS-affected people were abandoned overnight by friends, had lost their houses, all their insurance and jobs. Homophobia and stigmatization encouraged the feelings of "denial" of the disease even in the HIV-positive people themselves who in turn purposely claimed their sero-negative status, refused to undergo any HIV test. Actual diagnosis was kept hidden even before family members including parents. Denial of the disease was more prominent among gays. Echoing Sheldon's feeling about it, Monette writes, "AIDS was rapidly turning into an inquisition in the gay community, as rife with terror and scapegoats as any launched by Rome. Does this one have it? Really? I heard it was his roommate. It gets so you can't be sick at all anymore. You hide colds, put Band-Aids on innocent bruises. You say you are fine when you want to scream" (82). These practices continued even after the death of AIDS patients as though HIV/AIDS itself became a synonym for panic and discrimination. Monette writes, "[...] I would hear at least every other week about the discreet death by AIDS of one or another rich man, the cause of death fudged on the certificate or otherwise unreported. Every gay man I know has stories of married bisexual men who died in the secret enclaves of family, town, church, and local GP, all without saying the "A" word. Even certain gay doctors, we heard, would blur a death certificate if the family was mortified enough" (308).

Reflecting on Roger's diagnosis that was kept hidden for sometime even before the parents, Monette introspectively writes: "I still have such conflicted feelings about hiding the diagnosis. What's privacy and what's denial? How much is guilt and the lingering self-hatred of the closet?"(81). He calls time with HIV/AIDS a "minefield of self-denial [...]" (87). However, as has been argued in Chapter-I, "denial" is the initial psychic norm to prove one's healthiness in opposition to unhealthiness. Of course, "The privacy issue surrounding AIDS engages vectors of the nightmare that make it different from every other medical crisis" (81).

Roger's sexual orientation and diagnosis could not be kept private for long. When Roger was sure of succumbing to HIV/AIDS, he finally told his father Al that he was gay. This revelation coupled with the knowledge of his two sons (Sheldon and Roger) being gay had thrown Al into a terrible depression. Al couldn't look Paul in the eye for a year and a half, couldn't speak his name or enter their house. However, Paul faced it with dignified courage. He accepted Roger's diagnosis of AIDS "not as a death sentence but rather as a life challenge" (80). He kept vigil for months together for Roger. He kept awake for many nights. Monette writes, "Waking teaches you pain" (342). To keep Roger alive under medical care, Paul spent almost all his savings in the bank after the full utilization of medical insurance cover of Roger who lost his wealthy clients following the disclosure of his infection with HIV/AIDS. With intense love and resolute care he left no stone unturned to save his lover Roger who suffered painfully from lesions, PCP, blindness, dementia and cryptococcal meningitis and was frequently confined to wheel chair, bed and hospital room at the UCLA Medical Center. It was through Paul's efforts that Roger was put on the AZT drug. Finally all his pains and care proved in vain as Roger died, that too, during his brief absence. However, Paul's constant concern for Roger had changed the anti-gay and heterosexual mindset of Al. In the last night of Roger's life, Al made a declaration about Paul in the hospital: "'This boy took care of him like a mother'" (341). This feeling can also easily be aroused in any reader, only because Monette treats HIV/AIDS like a leveller in his narrative scheme.

This was an avowal of gay love at a time when gay identity was under siege for its erasure. This avowal has been transformed into affirmation through references to the ancient Greek history with its central stress on free homosexuality. For example, Al viewed Paul's relationship with Roger thus: "'You boys are the best friends I've ever seen,' he said. 'You're like Damon and Pythias'" (318). This latter remark is explained by Monette: "A century after Socrates, Pythias was condemned to death in Syracuse but wished to go home and settle his affairs. Damon, his friend, took his place in jail, agreeing to be executed if Pythias didn't return. Of course he returned, and the tyrant who'd condemned him was so moved by the friendship that he released them both. This is not a myth" (318).

Greece has always been significant for a gay man who seeks his personal and historical identity in Greek characters. HIV/AIDS provides an opportune though fatal occasion for Monette to intensify his search for gay roots. Before Roger's diagnosis they visited Greece. Paul sentimentalized their visit:

> [...] the moment we set foot in Greece I was home free. Impossible to measure the symbolic weight

of the place for a gay man [...] about the homoerotic side [...]. The ancient soil becomes peopled with warrior brothers equal to fate [...]. The source of such heroics is buried very deep [...].

But you find that your first bewildered erotic connection at fourteen stays with you, since most of the rest of gay history lies in shallow bachelors' graves. [...] I swept across the Aegean at a fever pitch. [...] .

[...] Athens [...] was brisk with the winds of early summer, and the grass was thick in the *agora,* where Socrates had held forth. We drove to Delphi across the Theban plain [...] where Apollo slew Python [...].

[...]. We were, however, the most unreconstructed romantics, fanatic after our fashion [...].

[...]. When I ran in the grassy stadium high on the mountain where the Pythian Games were held, their heroes sung by Pindar, I knew I was poised at the exact center of my life. I belonged at last to a brotherhood where body and spirit were one. [...] In the pitch of the moment it seemed to me that Roger and I and our secret brothers were heir to all of it.

[...] ancient places "confirm" a person, uniting a man to the past and thus the future. Confirmed was just how I felt by the Greek idea. Hopeless romance: they kept slaves, their women were powerless, they sacrificed in blood. But a gay man seeks his history in mythic fragments, random as blocks of stone in the ruins covered in Greek characters, gradually being erased in the summer rain. We have the poems of Sappho [...]. Fragments

> are all you get. You jigsaw the rest with your heart.
>
> [..]
>
> [...] the ruins of ancient Thera [...] in 1500 B.C. gave Plato his myth of Atlantis [...] had [...] a gymnasium with an outdoor court [...] where the boys danced naked to Apollo. There are inscriptions along the walls, erotic poems to the boys [...].
>
> [...] You must discover the pagan on your own; it's not in the books. As to where a man finds his ancestors, the longing is diffuse till you come to a place where they spring full-blown. [...] The echo of the ancient image, warrior or monk is in you. (20-23)

Socrates, Plato, Pindar and Sappho belong to the ancient Greek's martial, fatalistic, philosophical and predominantly homosexual culture. Sappho, the poetess of Lesbos Island in the Aegean Sea was a lesbian. Monette also considers Roger to be a Greek:

> "Paul, we have to accept our fate," said Rog, firm and unsentimental. "There's no other choice."
>
> "But I can't," I whined, and I meant I *won't*. Yet even as I said it, it struck me how Greek Roger's attitude was. [...] I still wanted Greece to be sunny and exalted, with white stone ruins and statues of gods so perfectly human they breathed. [...] I wasn't equipped for the tragic design of fate. (220)

Monette historicizes gay identity to legitimize and naturalize it in a mandatorily heterosexual society. HIV/AIDS has been an occasion that befits such historicization that, in turn, vouches for the justification of author's warlike assertion of being gay. Monette shows the spirit of a warrior fighting the disease, fighting against moral, medical and juridical establishments of the society that targeted only homosexuals for victimization in the epidemic and in doing so tries to liberate beleaguered gay and HIV-positive identities.

Monette starts with how gay warriors are produced in the process of the systemic interpretation of gays in relation to HIV/AIDS: "The fact is, no one knows where to start with AIDS. [...] At first you are equipped with a hundred different amulets to keep it far away. Then someone you know goes into the hospital, and suddenly you are at high noon in full battle gear. They have neglected to tell you that you will be issued no weapons of any sort. So you cobble together a weapon out of anything that lies at hand, like a prisoner honing a spoon handle into stiletto. You fight tough, you fight dirty, but you cannot fight dirtier than it" (2). In order to strengthen his stand as a rebel against the forces denigrating gays infected with HIV/AIDS that was then used as both pretext and reason for stigmatization of homosexuals in general, he states his narrative intention: "The magic circle my generation is trying to stay within the borders of is only as real as the random past. Perhaps the young can live in the magic circle, but only if those of us who are ticking will tell our story. Otherwise it goes on being *us* and *them* forever, built like a wall higher and higher, till you no longer think to wonder if you are walling it out or in"(6). The magic circle is the metaphor for the illusion of health. This can also be taken as a sort of literary manifesto concerning HIV/AIDS on the part of the writer who is assertive enough to write with candour about his own experiences of the disease in its social and cultural milieu. There is a note of militancy in his assertion.

All along the book Monette, despite being HIV positive himself, has demonstrated his fighter's instinct in grappling with the problems of his AIDS-affected gay lover Roger, since he believes, "Warriors in pitched battle do not make their last will; they become it"(75). Looking back at the "passive" battle of HIV-positive people against discrimination and stigmatization, Monette laments: "I wish my fellow warriors hadn't lost the first four or five years bogged down by homophobia and denial. [...] It will be recorded that the dead in the first decade of the calamity died of our indifference" (18). He rationalizes to the point of refusing to accept blindly the American accusation theory concerning HIV/AIDS that was then targeting Africans as the sources and vectors of the disease: "The Africa connection was beginning to be in the news, with figures so pandemic the mind rejected the parallel. It was still only five thousand gay men, and nobody knew how long they had, maybe years. Cases that died in a month were something else; there was nobody fighting" (19). Monette's inexorable will to fight can also be seen when at one point he insists that those who claim for themselves seronegativity status for fear of being stigmatized are actually HIV positive people in denial. Monette wants those people to be tested compulsorily:

> There is such infinite variety about the way people tell you their negative status. Some are openly full of remorse and feel they have failed you.
>
> [...]
>
> Some hoot with excitement and forget you might not be as thrilled as they. I have friends who will not be tested at all because they know how shamefully glad they'll be. Their gut instinct is they're negative, so who are they trying to kid? They are always the first to tell you to stop being so AIDS-related. *Lighten up,* they say.
>
> [...] I want the two million-or the five million, depending on whose scenario piques your fancy-to have themselves tested and know, so I will have people to talk to. [...] I want to tap into

> the rage of the positives so we can throw buckets of sheep's blood on the White House lawn and spit in the faces of cops with yellow gloves. (164-65)

Here Monette the AIDS rebel assumes an angry AIDS activist position. When AIDS drug was not made available to patients because of procedural delay at the bureaucratic level, Monette's message was that everyone must start demanding the medical privileges such as drugs, because the system wasn't out to cut the red tape. He writes, "Indeed, red tape *was* - and largely still is - the system" (166).

This is also evident in the last part of the book when people sympathized with Monette with a note of fatalism. They said that how painful it was on the part of Paul to have a friend Roger in the "late" stages of AIDS. To these gestures the author retorted, "'There is no early or late,' [...]. 'There's only how much you fight it'" (269).

Regardless of sexual orientation or preference, any sensible reader of any gender, race, ethnicity and nation cannot help liking Monette's book dealing with the story of great gay love. Monette's book leaves a lasting impression that homosociality is natural, sacred and perhaps desirable. It is a bold pathfinder in its effective attempt to subvert the dominant notion of HIV/AIDS as permanently invalidating "gay identity." Monette proves that despite and because of HIV/AIDS, the infected can live as "positively" as the healthy, and gay identity can be meaningfully productive and perpetually retainable. Thus, he anticipates the movement of gay identity from the margin to the center of heterosexual matrix even through deadly odds for naturalization and normativization. The book serves as a lasting memorial to, or a perennial reminder of "positivity" and not negativity of HIV-positive people.

The "positivity" is nothing but the recuperative and meaningfully creative or productive engagement with "identity" that HIV/AIDS has caused, even though it may also be "passive" due to impending death. This is seen in *This Wild Darkness: The Story of My Death* (1996), an HIV/AIDS autobiography written under the prime obsession with his own death by sixty-five-year-old Harold Brodkey who was then given constant care by his wife Ellen Schwamm. Brodkey was diagnosed with HIV/AIDS by Barry Hartman, his doctor at New York Hospital in the spring of 1993 when he developed pneumocystis carinii pneumonia (PCP), suffocation and immobility, breathed through a tube in his nose, was confined to either wheel chair or bed and was hospitalized. He described his feeling of that moment thus: "This is how my life ended. And my dying began" (4). This experience of living through dying of HIV/AIDS continued till the late fall of 1995 when Brodkey wrote:

> I am at the end of the list of AIDS drugs to take. I wake frightened now; it is a strange form of fright—geometric, limited, final.
>
> Being ill like this combines shock—*this time I will die*—with a pain and agony that are unfamiliar, that wrench me out of myself. It is like visiting one's funeral, like visiting loss in its purest and most monumental form, this wild darkness, which is not only unknown but which one cannot enter as oneself. Now one belongs entirely to nature, to time: identity was a game. [...] Memory, so complete and clear or so evasive, has to be ended, has to be put aside [...]. It is death that goes down to the center of the earth, [...] and then to the curved ends of the universe [...].
>
> Call it the pit, the melodramatic pit: the bottomless danger in the world is bottomed with blood and the end of consciousness. Yet I don't wake [...] angrily prepared to fight or to accuse. (171-72)

Living with HIV/AIDS that erases "identity," memory,

and the will to fight or to accuse has been compared with "funeral," "wild darkness," centripetal death, "the pit" or hell and "the end of consciousness." It is also expressed thus: "At times I cannot entirely believe I ever was alive, that I ever was another self, and wrote - and loved or failed to love.[...] Oh, I can comprehend a shutting down, a great power replacing me with someone else (and with silence), but this inability to have an identity in the face of death - I don't believe I ever saw this written about in all the death scenes I have read or in all the descriptions of old age. It is curious [...] how my memories no longer apply to the body in which my words are formed" (172-73). This identity crisis caused by HIV/AIDS justifies the gloomy title of the book that focuses on Brodkey's own life-in-death experience.

Unlike Monette, Brodkey always accepts his HIV-positive state without rage, since he understands, "when you have AIDS, you're hospital material. The terminology is distinctive: you will die of 'complications from AIDS.' [...] Whoever you are, your biological identity now occupies a thin cage with prowling, opportunistic diseases. AIDS is not phallocentric, not homocentric, not picky in the least about its carrion; it is in the service of the grandeur of opportunism" (43).

This passivity stems from the acceptance of HIV/AIDS as heterosexual disease. The book is written in the 1990s when HIV/AIDS had been largely the epidemic of the "dominant" heterosexual community. Moreover, Brodkey himself was heterosexual by orientation, even though his "adventures in homosexuality took place largely in the 1960s and '70s [...]" (1). He had then visited gay bathhouses, had lived and had occasional sex with two men named Douglas and Charlie. Brodkey's recreational, casual homosexuality was "acquired" from his upbringing.

After the death of his mother Ceil who travelled alone from near Leningrad (in Russia) to Illinois (in the

US) in the 1920s, his father Max Weintrub, an illiterate, semiprofessional prizefighter sold two-year old Harold to relatives -the Brodkeys -for three hundred dollars. Harold got an adoptive father in Joe Brodkey and an adoptive mother in Doris Brodkey who was a cancer patient. They used to live in a small Midwestern town called Alton and later moved to St. Louis.

Harold Brodkey was sexually abused. Talking about Joe's paedophilia he writes, "Anyway, the major drama of my adolescence was that my adoptive father, Joe Brodkey, who was ill with heart trouble [...] assailed me every day for two years, sexually—twice a day, every morning and every evening, when I was twelve and thirteen. He had nothing else to do, really. He was ill. We were not the same blood. I am being very shy. He never succeeded in entering me, but it was somewhat scary and sweaty" (58). Doris asked Harold to cooperate with Joe in his sexual act with "he-can't-live-without-you things [...]" (58). She even cautioned Harold, "'If I were you, I'd learn to keep my mouth shut'" (59). She advised, "'You never seem nice if you have to say no'" (59). The author confessed nothing, complained to no one about what he felt about the sexual assaults then. Rather, Joe and Doris both were interested in "this *love* thing" (59). This was how the author was initiated into homosexuality. As Brodkey puts it, "my identity was at the moment caught. Either of my parents would have killed the other for me" (59). This explains why the author later in his life briefly visited homosexual bathhouses and lived with two gays. This became the most important point of reference in the writer's story of death, since Harold believed that he was infected by Charlie who later died of HIV/AIDS. He writes, "I think he was the one who gave it to me" (143). In trying to locate the source of his infection in his homosexual experiences, Harold is simply confirming his heterosexist notion of HIV/AIDS as a gay disease.

Brodkey's "straight" orientation is also revealed when

he writes, "I was never accepted as gay by anyone, including someone who lived with me and claimed to be a lover. [...] Toward the end of my experience of homosexuality, before I met Ellen, I underwent the most outrageous banishment to a role of sheer, domineering, hated and worshipped masculinity" (29-30). Ellen Schwamm with her children left her first husband to be with Harold. Ellen was also a novelist. Their marital love was self-giving and self-exceeding as well. For example, the detection of Harold's HIV-positive status filled Ellen with depression, since she was HIV-negative and hence felt separated from him. She exclaimed, "Oh, I don't want to be clear. I want to have it, too" (34). Even though the author is sceptical about his wife's emotion, he at this point confesses, "She wanted to die of what I was going to die of" (35).

Ellen's great love and care for Harold at home after his refusal to be in hospital is a life-giving experience for the author who writes about his wife, "[...] she is father and mother and wife and husband and daughter and son; she is herself and the me-of-the-vanished-years" (159). He was mostly living "because of Ellen [...]" (164). Their deep relationship continued uninterrupted for fifteen years till Harold died of HIV/AIDS in January 1996. This is why the book has appropriately been dedicated to his wife Ellen who is hailed by the author as "my light" on the dedication page of the book. Ellen was the light in Harold's life of darkness. The valorization of long-lasting opposite-sex love in a family situation points to Brodkey's intrinsic heterosexuality, despite his picture of his premarital bisexuality that is described thus, "I could offer a list of the men I have had (or the women I have had)"(28). Thus, Brodkey's book has a heterosexual perspective that generally serves to promote the notion of HIV/AIDS as a gay disease. Hence, the book is surcharged with sombreness in its depiction of the impact of HIV/AIDS on personal identity.

Once individual identity is invaded by HIV/AIDS,

there is no escape, no fighting back. Brodkey writes, "The fundamental situation is all clarity and obscurity: a doomed boxing match with a submicroscopic virus that can have no real sense of the identity of its opponent and yet which, in its micro-ignorance, must win. It eats you alive" (63). Living with HIV/AIDS amounts to silence and nothingness. Death is always imminent. Brodkey writes, "Death itself is soft, softly lit, vastly dark. The self becomes taut with metamorphosis [...]. Living, one undergoes one metamorphosis after another [...] but they are continuous and linked. This one is a stillness and represents a sifting out of identity and its stories, a breaking off or removal of the self, [...]" (24). His sense of 'spoiled' identity is seen in his response to Ellen when she requests him for a kiss, "'Ellen, I'm filthy with AIDS. I have viruses crawling in me, hideous - hideous wrigglers. I smell to high heaven. I don't want to kiss anyone [...]'" (118).

Even authorial or autobiographical identity is in question, since according to Harold, "The trouble with death-at-your-doorstep is that it is happening to you. Also, that you are no longer the hero of your own story, no longer even your narrator. Barry was the hero of my story and Ellen the narrator. The tale was of my death amid others' lives—like a rock in a garden" (68). The inherent paradox in this self-conscious announcement is shockingly juxtaposed with the authorial practice when he says, "And I am still writing, as you see. I am practicing making entries in my journal, recording my passage into nonexistence. This identity, this mind, this particular cast of speech, is nearly over" (169). These contradictions apparently stem from the stifling awareness of the unpredictable cessation of thinking, writing and life due to HIV/AIDS at any moment. However, the writing is testament to his fact of living with HIV/AIDS. This understanding is reflected as Harold writes, "I exist. I matter *now.* [...] the writing is an anodyne [...]" (110).

This once again stands in sharp contrast to his initial

reaction to the disease, "When Barry said I had AIDS, I said I didn't believe him. [...] I was embarrassed and shamed [...]" (4). The cause of this denial can be seen in the light of analysis given in Chapter-I. Doctor Barry assured the writer that after the Pneumocystis cleared up, he had the possibility of a few years of life. However, the writer's gut feeling then was that it would be embarrassing to live with "The stigma. Incontinence. (Would I have to wear a diaper?) Blindness" (6). An HIV- positive patient in the process is practically reduced to "a lousy conversation piece" (44). Person with HIV/AIDS is made a "mockery of everything one was before—mentally and physically, socially and erotically, emotionally and politically" (162). Harold fails to reciprocate the love of his wife, since he feels, "[...] I am an object of charity" (117). He also knows pretty well the social and cultural effects of HIV/AIDS. He writes, "The separation from society, the political marginalization and the financial thefts, the attacks to see what can be stolen from you, and the indignity—including social indignity—of AIDS suggest a partial, sometimes fluorescent and linoleumed version of the death camps"(44). This unpleasant state of affairs together with consequent suffering associated with HIV/AIDS induces Barry to advise Harold to keep his disease a secret. The writer also understands that "[...] to die of AIDS is to die outside a tradition, in a silence of sorts" (77).

However, as a writer Harold Brodkey rationalizes to keep his identity intact. He writes, "In the confused, muddled velocities of my mind was an editorial sense that this was wrong, that this was an ill-judged element in the story of my life. I felt too conceited to have this death. [...] I took inside me the first stirrings of acknowledgment of AIDS, [...] with the different sense of aloneness" (6-7). The writer refuses to be seen as someone destined to be condemned, as someone arousing pity in others, including his wife Ellen and doctor Barry. He writes, "I suppose I had made up my mind to try not to be humiliated, and that involved my not being pitiable [...]" (9). Initially, Harold's disease was not disclosed to other members of his family, including their children, to his lawyer, agent, or friends. It was only confined to Ellen, Barry and hospital workers. Even then the over-acuteness of the sense of internalized stigma in him prevented Harold from chatting freely with women workers in the hospital. He writes, "I was shy and self-conscious, ashamed that my blood represented a risk" (72). However, Harold has his own reason for keeping his disease a secret: "I had no wish to put my [...] great helplessness on exhibit. I did not want my drowned, limp, whispering self magnified into anecdote. I did not want to be goaded into the effort of public behavior. (I could apologetically claim that I had no strength to show gratitude if people were kind.) The collective vigor of the people we were close to—well, if they should form a phalanx of wills, [...] then I would have to adopt their definitions of my predicament. It seemed too messy and difficult to speak of any of this, or to speak and omit this, or to ask Ellen to speak to everyone for me" (73).

Harold also faces his HIV-positive status with an audacious sense of humour as he equates his orphanhood with the disease that, being absolutely different, isolates him from his ancestral diseases. He writes, "[...] I was cut off from my family inheritance of fatal diseases—the strokes and high blood pressure and cancer and tumors of my ancestors" (23). Ruminating on his different medical fate Harold observes, "I felt a bit orphaned again, and [...] as if I had been invited, almost abducted, to a party, a somber feast [...], a feast of the seriously afflicted who yet were at war with social indifference and prejudice and hatred. It seemed to me that I was surrounded by braveries without number, that I had been inducted into a phalanx of the widely-alive-even-if-dying, and I felt honored that I would, so to speak, die in the company of such people" (23).

This is unmistakably the positive thinking of Harold

imaginatively identifying with people living with AIDS. This non-defeatist's impulse urged Brodkey to write in the *New Yorker* an essay on the subject of his own dying from AIDS. In fact, parts of this autobiography were published when he was alive. He disregarded Barry's strong recommendation for secrecy to avoid public humiliation and to live longer: "I'd rather be open about AIDS and scoff at public humiliation than feel the real humiliation of lying. I'd rather try to make this a death as much like any other as I can. Culture aims toward death, no matter what it says" (115). For Harold lying, denying and hiding are conservative, a bourgeois life style. This act of pretence shows that "One appreciates the urge to sanitize and control, the punitive framework and the denial of sexual authenticity" (29). Therefore, truth or honesty for the author is therapeutic, "a form of caress" (114). His candour about his HIV-positive status is "chiefly an objection to the world itself, a sort of challenge: *Let's see how you are going to lie to me now.* [...] I knew that Barry had been afraid of me, that he encouraged lying as a way to make things easier for the person with AIDS" (154). This soul-searching in the face of HIV/AIDS makes Harold feel happy: "It seems very strange to think one could enjoy one's death. Ellen has begun to laugh at this phenomenon. We know we are absurd, but what can we do? We are happy" (176).

However, Harold also shows resignation as he writes, "Death is a bore. But life isn't very interesting either. I must say I expected death to glimmer with meaning, but it does not. It's just there. I don't feel particularly alone or condemned or unfairly treated, but I do think about suicide a lot because it is so boring to be ill [...]" (152). Death is preferable to illness for him as he loses his sense of people. Finally, Harold realizes that HIV/AIDS is more real than theological actuality, "God is an immensity, while this disease, this death, which is in me, this small, rightly defined pedestrian event, is merely real, without miracle -or instruction" (177).

In the book ideas and feelings do not cohere and are unstable. In the text there is a disruption of sequentiality, is a kind of aporia. This incoherence is symbolic of split identity that HIV/AIDS has caused. As Brodkey rightly feels, "I am what is called a disconnector: some measurements of my condition are favorable and others are not, but they move in ways unrelated to one another when they should move conjointly" (163). The most amazing disconnection is how Ellen and their daughter remained uninfected with HIV/AIDS despite Brodkey's premarital exposure to the disease way back in 1977 when he, as his chaotic chronicle reveals, had his "last" homosexual relation. In fact, the book begins thus, "I have AIDS. [...] I have not been exposed since 1977, [...]" (1). It suggests that Harold had been infected with AIDS before 1977. Despite the disjunction between thoughts and feelings, a disjunction that eventually leads to rupture of linearity, Harold achieves liberation from the constraints and stereotypes of the notion of HIV-positive identity.

This liberation is ethical and energizing as well. This liberationist identity of an author is also found in the physician's autobiography titled *My Own Country: A Doctor's Story* (1994) by Abraham Verghese, an Indian doctor who specialized in infectious diseases. Without himself being infected with HIV/AIDS, he sees the disease from clinical and non-native perspectives. Unable to complete his medical education in Ethiopia (Africa) where he was born of expatriate Indian Christian parents, Verghese went to America where he worked as an orderly in hospitals and nursing homes for sometime. He then came to India where he passed all medical exams to go back again this time with Rajani Chacko, his newly married wife from India to the United States as a rookie doctor in 1980. He worked as a resident at East Tennessee State University in Johnson City where his wife also did her MBA, went then to Boston City Hospital to specialize in infectious diseases, again came back to Johnson City to be a teacher and clinician. The safe, rural, pastoral setting of Tennessee provided him a base for settling down. Verghese writes, "And instead of escalating goals, I wanted nothing more than to settle in one place and be a good physician. Stateless and roaming for so long, I wanted to put down roots" (46). He became a naturalized citizen of Tennessee, which he calls "my own country" (46). The country here stands for both nation state and rurality. Verghese was working as a staff at the Mountain Home Veterans Administration Medical Center and as a consultant at the adjacent community hospital called Johnson City Medical Center (popularly known as "the Miracle Center") at the same time. He was "THE DE FACTO AIDS expert in Johnson City even though there was no AIDS to see" (52). Initially his job was limited to giving public talks or media interviews on HIV/AIDS. However, before long, like "the umbilical cords" he was "fastened" (428) to eighty-plus HIV-infected people during his five-year stint in Johnson City. The pregnancy metaphor suggests how doctor Verghese was inseparably attached to HIV- positive people. As a physician, he played the crucial role of both a keen observer and an active participant "in a culture of disease, a small island in a sea of fear" (428).

On his permanent departure from Johnson City as an AIDS doctor on the first day of 1990, Verghese towards the concluding part of his narrative very touchingly writes: "I left my own country, my beloved Tennessee. Perhaps my perennial migrations, almost hereditary, are a way to avoid loss. With deep roots come great comforts. Yet deep attachments are the hardest to lose. Maybe that is why drifters avoid them" (427). The innate sense of deracination coupled with sudden detachment from his deep attachment to his HIV-positive patients fills Verghese with a sense of guilt: "I feel so guilty over this sense of liberation. I feel such pain when I think of their faces" (428). As he is on his way to Iowa to pursue scholarly research leaving behind Johnson City, he also feels, "Never before AIDS and Johnson City have I felt so close to love and pain, so connected to other people"(428).

Thus, the autobiography is written from the points of view of both an outsider and an insider. It also demonstrates how Verghese was in search of his identity, of his home, of his own country. His spiritual acceptance of his rootedness in his profession of treating persons living with HIV/AIDS with love can be seen when he generalizes his own perception of identification of a doctor with the patient: "I suppose every doctor at some point sees himself or herself reflected in the patient seated opposite, every doctor begins to ask what blind luck has resulted in being the *listener* and not the reciter of the horrid tale being told, what would it be like to be the patient?" (333). Verghese's message aims at breaking down the doctor's stereotypical role as privilege-seeker rather than caregiver. Likewise, he also attacks the pre-HIV/AIDS-era beliefs of the Western medical world in the absolutely certain comprehension and conquest of any disease and in the mastery over the human body. For him, these beliefs were the products "of unreal and unparalleled confidence, bordering on conceit [...]. Only cancer was truly feared, and even that was often curable. When the outcome of treatment was not good, it was because the host was aged, the protoplasm frail, or the patient had presented too late - never because medical science was impotent" (24). The challenge posed by HIV/AIDS to the canonical privilege of the medical science concerning disease has been discussed in Chapter-I. In this situation, Verghese's approach to his patient sounds pre-modern in its affiliation. However, it is practically appropriate. He treats the sick as the whole that includes their body, mind, soul, society and culture. This sense of holism requires homefeeling, oneness and personal touch with the ill who in turn develop a dignified sense of belonging with the world.

This is seen when Verghese deconstructs the

conventional paradigm of the country-city dichotomy in HIV/AIDS discourse. His case study, on the one hand, indicates, "[...] infection with HIV in rural Tennessee was largely an *imported* disease. Imported to the country from the city. Imported by native sons who had left long ago and were now returning because of HIV infection" (395). On the other hand, he also observes, "[...] around Johnson City [...] were patients who lived [...] *and* acquired their infection in [...] the 'local-locals', [...]" (395). The "local-locals" were inhabitants of the Tri-cities namely Johnson City, Bristol and Kingsport that are considered the countryside of the US.

Verghese also de-categorizes HIV-positive classification such as homosexual, hemophiliac, Haitian, heroin addict, heterosexual, the innocent and the guilty. As he puts it, "Of course, the virus, unlike human beings, lacked all class prejudice" (251). He himself has proved it in his initial health education and public speaking efforts at the Connection (renamed later as New Beginnings), a gay bar in Johnson City. After his arrival in Johnson City as intern and resident, Verghese was familiar with gay bars, gay culture and bathhouses only through "reading" about them. That's why he writes, "I knew no *openly* gay man. I only knew the stereotype" (23). He then sensed that the stereotype might be untrue. In order to establish it, he ventured to visit the Connection in Johnson City, "a place where Jerry Falwell's pronouncement that homosexuals would 'one day be utterly annihilated and there will be a celebration in heaven' was taken as a self-evident truth" (56). He had the subconscious fear of himself being seen entering, leaving or staying in the Connection that was then visited by the police for surveillance. Despite the fear, he visited the gay bar along with Olivia Sells, the director of the local Red Cross to speak to gays on safe sex and on blood test for HIV. His speech inspired many gays who opted voluntarily for blood test. Verghese was surprised by the test results. He writes, "To my utter amazement, not one of the patrons of the Connection who obtained the test was infected with the virus" (69). This was in 1986 when in San Franscisco HIV/AIDS affected largely gay community. Verghese's findings disprove the orthodoxy surrounding the gays in relation to HIV/AIDS. All along the book, Verghese boldly downplays or resists the dominance of the stereotype.

He also demonstrates this through recounting the stories of his different HIV/AIDS patients who have a strong influence on him. The significant ones are the stories of Gordon, Ed Maupin and Bobby Keller, Fred Goodson and Otis Jackson, Vickie McCray vis-à-vis Clyde, Ethan Nidiffer, Luther Hines, Norman Sanger, and Will Johnson and Bess Johnson. These stories throw light on the people's perception of HIV/AIDS in small towns in America. They also focus on a doctor's quest for identity that eventually emerged out of Verghese's immersion in the affairs of HIV/AIDS both in the clinic or hospital and in his own home.

The story of Gordon is about a gay who had an honourable death from HIV/AIDS. Gordon's background was narrated to Verghese by Gordon's elder sister Essie Vines who was in her early forties, was working as a lab technician in a little hospital in Virginia. As a child, Gordon Vines was sickly and often suffered from croup, bronchitis and fits. Failing to pursue his studies at the University of Virginia due to lack of funds, Gordon worked together with Essie for sometime in an ammunition factory in Kingsport. Gordon was gay. However, Essie's feeling for her brother was different, "'[...]. I knew then that Gordon was gay. But I didn't have any special word for it, you understand? I didn't think too much about it, you know? He was just Gordon [...]. Even now, I can't think of him as gay. Gay may have been what he did, but it wasn't who he was. He was our Gordo before he was anything else'" (92). This is tacit acknowledgement and acceptance of gay identity in a family situation. Essie's version was that Gordon had a God-given talent, was capable of doing something different, something unique. Listening to similar stories from the families of gay men, Verghese is puzzled by the notion of the gifted talent of the homosexuals: "There was always the God-given talent that accompanied their God-given sexuality, always the special creativity and humor. This fascinated me. Was it part of the subconscious effort to compensate for their difference? Was the charm and talent as biologically determined as the sexuality?"(92).

Gordon was a prodigal son. He landed a job in Atlanta where he lived with John, a flight attendant for an airline. He frequently traveled to Mexico, Paris and New Orleans. Then Gordon disappeared for four years and hence was given up for lost. On Mother's Day he once called up his mother from Florida where he was living for many years with his male friends. There he got the diagnosis that he was HIV positive. He had two lovers who died of AIDS. Perhaps he got the virus from them. Unable to bear the pains of the disease, he finally returned home. He had fever, Kaposi's sarcoma lesion and pneumonia. He was looking pale with his cheeks collapsing onto the bone. He was hospitalized under the friendly care of Verghese at the Miracle Center in Tennessee. In fact, the nursing staff had been very friendly with Gordon. After he was discharged, some nurses from the Miracle Center travelled up to Blackwood, Norton (Virginia) to visit him. For sometime he worked as a hairdresser in a salon in a nearby town. However, he was very tired and sick. When Verghese told Gordon's parents that their son had AIDS, they did not accept it. Even after the death of Gordon, his mother did not talk about the disease, and his father always believed that his son died of stroke. However, despite his gay and HIV-positive status, Gordon had always been treated well by his family and medical professionals. Perhaps he was lucky enough not to be stigmatized. Only at the time of burial, A.J.Doochie Jones, the funeral service provider of Vines's family was scared to prepare the dead body of Gordon in his mortuary due to his deep belief in the possible transmission of HIV/AIDS through touch. However, George Wiseman gladly buried the body with conventional dignity and honor for the deceased.

The story of Ed Maupin and Bobby Keller is about what Verghese calls "the truck stop sex" (115). Ed Maupin was in his early forties, a diesel truck mechanic working for a trucking company in Abingdon in rural Tennessee. He had been married and was the father of three children who were all grown up. However, as Verghese narrates, "Ed was not bisexual, but gay. The marriage had been an attempt to conform but after many years his instinct for a sexual relationship with men had won out. For the last ten years Ed had lived in a steady relationship with Bobby Keller" (113). Bobby Keller worked as a salesperson in an Abingdon boutique. He was effeminate, a clown. He had been married and had fathered two children. He himself assessed his own identity thus: "'Lord knows I *tried* to be straight. I was having sex with Ed when I was seven. But I kept telling myself it was wrong, wrong, wrong, and so I got married to make me straight. Well all through my marriage I was tempted by men. Finally I just had to more or less admit to myself that there was no two ways about it. I was about as straight as a three-dollar bill'" (114).

The gay relationship between Ed and Bobby continued in spite of their heterosexual marriages that later on ended in divorce. Thereafter they lived together. Their instinct for sex with men drove them often to a truck stop where truckers heading down from the New York-Washington, D.C. branched off in different directions. There they had quick, anonymous sexual encounters. Bobby used to have frequent anal intercourse with the truckers who believed that their occasional partners from rural Abington were safe. Truckers who were not gay and did not like to pay for having sex with women usually preferred oral sex: "[...] most of what went on at the truck stop was oral sex" (115). Ed and Bobby engaged in unsafe sex practice that aroused anxiety in them. They came to Verghese to know for sure if they were infected with HIV. They were found to be HIV positive. Within a couple of weeks Ed had a bad pneumonia from HIV/AIDS and was hospitalized. He had serious breathing problem. Verghese's instruction to put Ed on the breathing machine was opposed by Bobby, who was doing what Ed desired. Ed's wish was not to be on machines. Now legally who would make decision for Ed? Whether Bobby or Ed's family? Bobby did not have any written note or living will from Ed in this regard. Ed's younger brothers expressed their decision: "'We are his family. We are legally responsible for him. We want you to do *everything* for him'" (223). Even as Verghese was listening to the decision of the family, he "watched Bobby's face crumble as he suddenly became a mere observer with no legal right to determine the fate of the man he had loved since he was seven years old. He was finally [...] an outsider" (223). When Ed died, a nurse remarked, "'Well, they're *all* going to die, aren't they? There's not much point to this'" (227). This made Verghese furious:

> I wanted to ask her what the 'point' was in the ninety-year-old patients that they played with in the unit for days until they were brain dead, all the while running up a huge bill that we, the taxpayers, would pay? Right at that moment there was a patient in the ICU whom we were sending up for dialysis three times a week when there was no hope of any other organ in the body recovering.
>
> I wanted to ask her if *she* was in the same boat, would she like an extra year of life, or would she opt to leave the world right away? And for that matter, weren't we ALL going to die one

> day? Did she think her job was to solely take care of immortals? (228)

Here is a doctor who crusades for the cause of HIV-positive people and gay identity as well. After the death of Ed, Bobby Keller joined the Tri-City AIDS Project (TAP), a community-based support group in Johnson City till he died from AIDS.

The TAP was formed by Fred Goodson who was a gay lover of Otis Jackson. Fred and Otis were two men in their late thirties. Both of them were from Tennessee. Fred studied in a college in Florida and worked for his master's in psychology at Madison in Wisconsin. Giving up a teaching position at a community college, eventually he joined his uncle's accounting business in Tennessee. Despite some heterosexual dating in his college days, he failed to continue his relationship with a girl, since he was gay. In Wisconsin he joined the Gay Liberation Front, became an activist and was involved with the Metropolitan Community Church (MCC) formed by a gay Pentecostal minister, Troy Perry who had written a book titled *The Lord Is My Shepherd and He knows I Am Gay*. Otis was trained as a cook, had worked for five years in the Castro District of San Francisco before he returned to Tennessee. They had "Tweedledum and Tweedledee sameness, a sense that they belonged to a gay community, that they subscribed to a defined gay aesthetic – at once together, at once defiant" (122). This gay couple had had sex with several people in the past. Fred had been to bathhouses in New York or Atlanta. Otis had several sexual encounters in San Francisco and in California. This was how they acquired HIV/AIDS. Fred had known enough about AIDS. Ever since he was diagnosed as HIV positive, he was interested in forming an AIDS support group. After several rounds of meeting with the coordinator of Tennessee AIDS Project, Fred succeeded in forming the TAP. Fred's sister Bettie Lee was also very supportive of both Fred and Otis. Despite Otis's reluctance, they used to hold regular meetings among the HIV-positive people to generate support and to devise ways to receive state and federal funds. At last Otis was bedridden and given morphine to have a peaceful death. Otis died in Fred's arms. However, in the funeral ceremony of Otis, the preacher said, "'Lord is merciful but we have to live with the consequences of our sins'" (379). This irritated Fred who then felt like strangling the preacher. Fred was doing well as an AIDS activist with TAP.

So was Vickie McCray with TAP. Her husband Clyde was a thirty-five-year-old truck driver. When she was told that her husband was HIV positive in the hospital, she came back home, impulsively loaded the gun, thought of shooting Clyde, her four-year-old son and twelve-year-old daughter and finally herself. However, her love for her children prevented her from doing this. By the time Vickie married Clyde out of her attraction to him, Clyde had been married twice. When Vickie was pregnant with her second child, Clyde was discovered to have slept with her unmarried sister who got pregnant later. She did not have a secured shelter and enough money to leave her husband.

Even though Clyde had so many different jobs, the money was never enough. He became an alcoholic. He then studied truck-driving in Florida to become a truck driver. He was working hard. There he started losing his weight and developed hiccups. Diagnosis revealed that he had AIDS. To Verghese's question if he had had sex with another man, Clyde's answer was emphatically positive: "'I've had sex with men' [...]. 'With Jewell, all the time'" (130). Jewell was a family friend and a married man. Vickie was surprised to hear this.

Clyde was obviously a bisexual. He was infected with HIV/AIDS and had also infected Vickie and her sister whose test reports were positive. However, their children were not infected. After learning about their HIV-positive status, her community, including her cousins and neighbors avoided them, did not even look at them. As Vickie puts it: "'You know people around here are so damn inquisitive they wouldn't hesitate to stop a funeral to ask what deceased the corpse!'"(140). Clyde wanted to go to church because of his sickness. Vickie's cousin had told the whole church about Clyde's disease and as a result, the church did not want him there. Vicikie had tolerated everything – her husband's sexual betrayal, disease and society's indifference. She had fought with them with compassion, forgiveness and with an indomitable spirit not to give in. Accepting Verghese's advice she finally joined Fred's support group TAP. Meanwhile Clyde died. Vickie became more active with TAP. She once went to church with a request to the preacher that the congregation should be told that she had AIDS. However, her children begged her not to do so. They feared that they might be stigmatized in school, in case their classmates who also went to the same church came to know about her infection. Vickie was visiting HIV-positive people every other day, looking after them. She spoke to Verghese about her newly found identity, "I have become a person I didn't know existed inside of me. [...] I'm now on the board of TAP! Can you believe it? An old country hick like me? I'm living my life to the fullest and thanking God for each day that I'm here. Life is so precious [...]. I'm more of a complete person that I ever was. [...] I am somebody. I'm happier now that I've been in a long time. I enjoy life more now'" (413). A new Vickie was shaped out of her involvement with activities pertaining to HIV/AIDS: "'I know that what I have is like a time bomb waiting to blow up in me and cause this terrible AIDS to begin. But I can't let it rule my life, get into my train of thought all the time and take away the best fight that my body possesses, and that is 'positive thinking.' I'm going to fight this disease with lots of laughter on account of, you know, it will boost my immune system'" (413). Vickie's experience as a housewife, as the head of the household, as a widow, as an AIDS patient and, finally, as an AIDS activist is really a story of assertion of identity and of affirmation of faith in oneself in the face of HIV/AIDS.

The story of Ethan Nidiffer reveals how HIV/AIDS causes panic among pharmacists and dentists. Ethan Nidiffer was in his late sixties and was an unmarried man. He was gay. For years four married men used to visit him to have him perform oral sex on them. He was HIV positive and Verghese's patient and later joined TAP. After the infection he found it difficult to get a dentist for his regular dental checkup, since dentists feared AIDS. In order to have a painful molar tooth pulled out, he tried with many dentists. Everybody refused, since he was HIV positive. Lastly he managed one dentist Dr.J to whom he did not disclose anything. After the tooth was extracted there was much bleeding. The blood splashed and spilled on to doctor's hands and eyeglasses. After the operation Ethan was asked to buy penicillin from the pharmacist.

The pharmacist who knew Ethan's HIV-positive status informed Dr.J over phone that he had just operated on an AIDS patient. This took Dr. J by panic. He called up Verghese to say: "'My wife and I...we have small children....I'm thinking of giving up dentistry altogether....I'd just as soon raise cattle or move away....If the Lord spares me, I swear I'll be a farmer or something else, but not dentistry....'"(301). He was crying thinking that he had got AIDS. Dr.J hadn't cut himself, had no open wounds at the time of operation. He was also wearing gloves. Even though Dr.J had little to fear, Verghese advised him to take barrier precautions such as wearing gloves and goggles for any dental operation. In addition to these things, he recommended two successive HIV tests in six weeks and six months to Dr.J. However, he entered into a heated argument with Ethan's pharmacist who rather interpreted the gross violation of his business ethics to keep the patient's identity a secret as his civic responsibility and, in addition, warned

Verghese that he did not want any more any of his AIDS patients. Of course, Verghese was aware that the pharmacists made huge profits by selling very expensive AZT to AIDS patients, had very often violated their ethics, had betrayed the confidence of the HIV-positive customers. AIDS patients were made to feel uneasy in the store. The moment an HIV/AIDS prescription was handed over to the pharmacist at the counter, it would be passed on to the other employees behind the counter. This would then be followed by complete silence. Everybody in the pharmacy would eye the patient who would be paying for the drug.

Luther Hines's is a story of the willpower of an AIDS patient. Luther Hines moved back from California to his home in Johnson City. He was HIV positive and almost without muscles on his bones because of the impact of the disease. His mother didn't want him. So too was his father who had a new wife. To all kinds of queries from Verghese, he was always aggressively defiant. For example, to the question of putting him in the hospital, his answer would be, "'What for? I'm not going to no hospital'" (377) To the question if he was staying with his parents, he responded, "'Why should I? I don't need them'" (377). To the question as to who was getting groceries and cooking for him, he shouted, "'I do. Okay? I do. I DON'T NEED ANYBODY'S HELP'" (377). He brushed aside the doctor's suggestion to join TAP. However, one day he spoke in the TAP meeting. He vehemently denounced his own parents, Dr. Verghese, persons with AIDS in general. He spoke nonstop and finally breezed out of the meeting. He had the indomitable will to survive. Despite his blindness from HIV/AIDS infection, he still moved out of his apartment, got rides to the mall, took cabs to the doctor's office, cursed the people he bumped into. He lived on his own and did not want to be in hospice, TAP and any social support group for HIV/AIDS. Verghese comments: "He had become my poster boy, a walking testament to how will and belief can make up for lack of muscle, how anger can overcome blindness" (421).

The story of Norman Sanger is about the courage and dignity of a hemophiliac who gets infected with AIDS. Norman Sanger was a personnel manager in a large coalmine. He was perhaps infected with HIV/AIDS in his usual visits to hemophilia camps for the infusion of anti-haemophilic factor. He came to know about his HIV-positive status later at a time when he was engaged to Claire, a poor widow with a son. He pleaded for postponement of their marriage. However, Clair knowingly married Norman despite his haemophilia and HIV-positive status. They had been living for two years. However, Norman developed weight loss, fatigue and candidiasis. He was administered AZT, to which he responded dramatically for sometime. He was never worried about the issues of stigma, secrecy and prejudice concerning his infection, had never been in self-pity, despair and fear of death. For him, HIV/AIDS "was a disability to be worked around, to be negotiated and overcome" (336). Verghese writes, "Norman had no fear of death; death was something that I and all my other patients seemed to dread. It was the very thing that made AIDS so frightful, the *essence* of AIDS: the fact that it was a uniformly fatal disease. But this seemed to hold no fear for Norman" (338).

Verghese is even scared of the smell of HIV/AIDS. He can very well identify "[...] the faint and familiar scent of AIDS [...] a smell that still fills me with dread" (339). As for Norman, he always kept insisting, "'I want to be remembered for having had dignity. For courage. Sometimes it is so tough...'" (340). His grit and equanimity moved Verghese who violating the doctor's code of conduct before a patient cried in front of Norman. He writes, "[...] I felt ashamed for crying. What kind of message did it convey when you broke down in front of your patient? Certainly not message of hope. I prayed he did not misinterpret my crying as a sign that the end was very near" (342). Bleeding profusely Norman died a painful death in the absence of Verghese. Claire had no understanding of the disease and had always believed in her husband's recovery. Norman's death taught Verghese the lesson of giving a comfortable death to HIV/AIDS patients in their last hours through administering morphine. He writes, "Norman's death increased my resolve to be a presence at the bedside when I could. And I would carry morphine with me always, have it ready at each bedside, at moment's notice, ready to disconnect the head from the body's anguish" (372). This shows that euthanasia or mercy killing, be it legal or illegal, is ethical and desirable for Verghese.

The story of Will and Bess Johnson is about HIV infection through blood transfusion. Will Johnson was in his early fifties. He was on the board of directors at the University of Kentucky where he also chaired one of its foundations. Immediately after attending the funeral of his friend, he had a massive heart attack in the cemetery. He was rushed to nearby Bluepark hospital, Virginia. He was later airlifted to Duke University Medical Center for bypass surgery. After the surgery Will bled profusely and was given lots of blood from a blood bank at Duke. Four weeks after his surgery he experienced fever, sore throat, lymph node enlargement and fatigue. He contracted HIV through blood transfusion. Will had subsequently infected his wife Bess. After they were infected with HIV/AIDS, their primary concern had been confidentiality. Will was well known to everybody in Kentucky. Moreover, they had an adult son and daughter. To keep their infection a secret in their hometown, their local doctor Sarah Presnell had sent them to Dr Verghese who was in Tennessee. Will and Bess feared that disclosure might earn them a bad name, stigma and discrimination. Will knew that AIDS meant gay and sin in popular perception. Hence, they believed that the new place other than their hometown would be suitable for them to keep their infection a secret.

The plight of the Johnsons deeply affected Verghese, "Was it easier for me to sympathize and identify with this beautiful couple because they were *not* gay, *not* intravenous drug users? Because they reminded me of my parents? Will Johnson had at one point used the words "innocent victim" when describing his and his wife's situation. I had wanted to interrupt him and say that *all* victims of this virus were innocent" (250).

For him, the implication of the word "innocent" was that "everyone else out there with HIV who did not get it by a blood transfusion was 'guilty'" (250). At this point, Verghese scientifically analyses why at the early stage of HIV/AIDS the metaphor of "guilt" had always been associated with gays and Africans in North America. In those years, HIV- positive males outnumbered females: "And in all sexual acts, whether gay or straight, it is the male that is always *injecting* semen, injecting a secretion into a partner, whether a woman or another man. For these reasons, gay men had been disproportionately affected by the virus. 'AIDS' in a man had come to mean 'gay' until proven otherwise" (251). For the dominant heterosexual world, there would be no AIDS without gay men. Africans were also attributed to be "guilty" by the journalists whose theory was that female circumcision coupled with traumatic and indiscriminate copulation among Africans helped transmit HIV and other STDs. This in turn helped shape the Africanness of the disease in the American cultural imagination. In fact nobody is to blame. Verghese declassifies all HIV/AIDS categories. By taking up the cause of HIV/AIDS he himself increasingly felt a sense of isolation from his medical fraternity, friends, and even from his wife. The association of the term "HIV/AIDS" had tarnished his reputation as a doctor. He felt as "guilty" as the kind of people he cared for. For this reason, he developed equation with the Johnsons: "Perhaps *this* was why I was so drawn to the Johnsons, the 'innocents': they were an affirmation of *my* self-worth, of *my* innocence" (253).

After a thorough medical checkup, Verghese concluded that Bess was asymptomatic and would live longer than her husband. Will was keen on maintaining secrecy even as Verghese was worried about their painful aloneness in their preference for secrecy. However, Will's feeling was different: "We are *not* alone. The one unshakable presence in our life is Christ. I personally think this thing, this virus, is from hell, from the devil himself. It is not from god. Nor do I believe God 'let it happen'" (291). In the hospital Will had a vision of Jesus Christ Who was assuring him that He would be fighting for him. On recommendation from Verghese, Will went once again to Duke for better treatment with AZT therapy. However, their secrecy could not be maintained any longer. They finally revealed their HIV-positive status to their son and daughter. Some days later Will slipped into coma and died. In a few months the brokenhearted Bess also died when AZT failed to work on her.

Through these stories, Verghese shows that a doctor is shaped and known by the patients he or she treats and that identity of a caring and good HIV/AIDS physician is as complex as the disease itself. Here is a doctor who rationally tries to understand homosexuality through the interaction with his gay patients. For Verghese homosexuality is not a nurtured or learned behavior. It is genetically present at birth. This is based on his experience with his gay AIDS patients: "So many gay men have told me how from the moment they were aware of their sexuality, they knew it was directed at men, not women" (59). In trying to explain to his wife at home, Verghese also reveals his understanding of gayness. In response to his stories of his gay patients, his wife retorted, "'Are you sexually attracted to the gay men?'"(142). His answer was in the negative and was followed by an explanation, " '[...] some of the sexual activity of gay men, their sexual drive, the number and variety of partners, the ready possibility of anonymous sex, might represent what *all* men want, except that they can't get women to agree'"(143). For Verghese, gays are "more representative of *men* than heterosexual men [...]" (142). Concerning sexual identity Verghese has also an important message to share:

> Why was it that *anonymous* sex, not just casual sex, rarely happened between men and women, only between men? Was it because the *woman* was the gatekeeper? Because *she* was less inclined to anonymous or casual sex? But a man, whether gay or straight, given his druthers, was quite capable of anonymous sex, could find it thrilling. I had never known a bar or club in any country that I had lived in where I could go and be *sure* of a sexual encounter with a woman - not without a monetary transaction. Did the prolific sexual activity of a gay bathhouse in its heyday, the anonymous sex, the multiple partners, the group sex, simply represent what *all* men were capable of if they had willing partners? Was this what a man would do if the gatekeeper were removed? (237).

Perhaps these questions raised by a heterosexual doctor would always remain rhetorical.

Verghese also writes about the fear of HIV/AIDS at home. When he wanted to share his experience of HIV/AIDS patients with his wife Rajani at home, he had only himself to partake in his empirical knowledge: "AIDS had become a mistress that took me away from home and that I could not introduce in conversation when I was at home" (288). Each time he was raising any thing concerning HIV/AIDS before Rajani, "her expression changed from concern and anxiety to [...] inscrutability. [...] she swallowed her fear, said nothing [...]" (75). A needlestick injury that once compelled him to perform occasional safe sex and frequent abstinence from sex with his wife for some months together till his HIV-test results were negative made him realize "how much fear she lived with; how it, indeed, filled her days while I was off playing hero" (75). Even his father asked him, "'Do you wear gloves when you touch them?'" (168). Despite Verghese's explanation that one cannot get HIV/AIDS from touch, his father cautioned him, "'[...]. Don't take chances'" (168). Verghese then felt, "I seemed to be living in a separate world which those who had not been touched by the disease could not enter. I felt [...] alone and unclean, chastened by my father's attitude" (168). Despite these, Verghese finds his identity in transforming his profession into mission. HIV/AIDS had entered into his unconscious mind, since it appeared time and again in his dream. He writes, "[...] I had a dream in which once again I contracted HIV. The dream recurred so often – always in different form – I thought of it as the 'infection' dream" (373). In his story, Verghese tries to challenge the phobic notion of HIV/AIDS.

3

Hegemonic American HIV/AIDS Fiction

This chapter and the chapter that follows it propose to consider the complex question of identity in some selected American HIV/AIDS fiction.

The exactness of effects of HIV/AIDS is difficult to imagine. As Thomas Yingling correctly states, "Inscribed since its appearance as profoundly unimaginable, as beyond the bounds of sense, the AIDS epidemic is almost literally unthinkable in its mathematical defeat of cognitive desire" (38). Therefore, while fictionalizing the paradoxical experience of HIV/AIDS in art, artists set some agendas or perspectives. The novelists' agendas are either to support or to question the ideology that underlies the cultural imagination of the epidemic. In this way, the writers seek to validate HIV-positive identities (such as gay, IV-drug user, haemophiliac, transfusion patient, guilty, innocent, African and so on), even if these identities are formed rightly or wrongly through the inscriptions of myths or interpretations. In so doing, they prevent HIV-positive people from being treated as nonexistent categories.

The novelists' perspectives in depicting the understanding of HIV/AIDS in their works may belong broadly to either hegemonic convention or counter-hegemonic practice. In the hegemonic convention, the HIV-positive people are portrayed in an intimidating way that arouses either sympathy, disgust (stigma) or fear. They are shown as fatalistic. They accept without any resentment or protest what happens to them or is in store for them. They face stigma stoically. This convention stresses self-abjection and non-identity on the part of the HIV- positive people.

It is challenged by counter-hegemonic practice that always deals with affirmation of identity. Counter-hegemonic HIV/AIDS narrative celebrates fighter's instinct in HIV-positive people. It is interventionist and demystifying. It subverts the dominant notion. It questions the social structures of stigma. It is activist in spirit. As Douglas Crimp in his essay "AIDS: Cultural Analysis/ Cultural Activism" puts it, "art *does* have the power to save lives, and it is this very power that must be recognized, fostered, and supported in every way possible. But if we are to do this, we will have to abandon the idealist conception of art. We don't need a cultural renaissance; we need cultural practices actively participating in the struggle against AIDS. We don't need to transcend the epidemic. We need to end it" (7). Counter-dominant literature recognizes that HIV/AIDS is, as has been shown in Chapter-I, partly social and linguistic constructions. Therefore, it provides a moot platform for its readers to always interrogate the interpretative communities around and the representational meanings of the epidemic. This is aptly described by Paula A. Treichler who writes, "The name AIDS in part *constructs* the disease and helps make it intelligible. We cannot therefore look 'through' language to determine what AIDS 'really' is. Rather, we must explore the site where such determinations *really* occur and intervene at the point where meaning is created: in language" (11). The novels that would be discussed in this chapter and the next chapter, by and large, explore the multiple social locations of the disease, and investigate how these sites eventually contribute to the multiple identities of the sick. Of course, in almost all HIV/AIDS fiction the above two motifs at times overlap.

This chapter attempts to focus on the issue of HIV-positive identity in four novels that belong to the dominant convention. The novels chosen for the purpose are M. E. Kerr's *Night Kites* (1986), Gloria D. Miklowitz's *Good-bye Tomorrow* (1987), Alice Hoffman's *At Risk* (1988) and Penny Raife Durant's *When Heroes Die* (1992).

Hegemonic constructions of disease, which represent illness as negation or loss of selfhood, frequently adopt the melodramatic mode, since they heighten the sense of shock, grief and self-accusation that sickness is supposed to elicit. This is especially so if the disease in question is stigmatized, like AIDS. One of the commonest scenarios is the family melodrama, where disease destroys the family's happiness and stability by unexpectedly striking one of its members, usually the one most loved. The above novels are good examples of this.

M.E.Kerr in her *Night Kites* (1986) focuses primarily on the moving saga of twenty-seven- year-old young man who is gay and subsequently has AIDS. The young man's plight is narrated by his seventeen-year-old younger brother who is heterosexual. In fact, the novel is written from the point of view of the younger brother. It uses first-person and third-person narration. Kerr juxtaposes homosexuality with heterosexuality and projects the former as a 'diseased' behaviour and the latter as a 'healthy' feeling. This binary opposition is in harmony with the cultural understanding of HIV/AIDS in America in the 1980s when the novel was written. She thus buttresses the hegemonic notion.

The Hudd family in New York includes Peter Rudd, his younger brother Erick Rudd and their parents. The novel explicitly depicts heterosexual relationship between Eric and his girlfriend Nicki Marr. The frequent reference to Edgar Allen Poe's romantic poem "Annabel Lee" that is about the immutability of heterosexual love also suggests that Kerr's is a dominantly straight world. Kerr introduces homosexuality only in the eighth chapter of the novel, when Pete in one of his trips to France with his friend Jim Stanley suffers from dysentery, is hospitalized and subsequently tests positive for AIDS. Pete's diagnosis with AIDS has a traumatic impact on his father who, while cautioning Eric not to disclose his brother's sickness to anyone, also feels, "'We just have to think about Pete. We're not going to judge him. We're going to support him'" (88). Here, Kerr evokes the HIV/ AIDS narrative convention of eventual non-judgmental acceptance of the infected by the family members despite their heterosexual mindset.

In a conversation with Erick, Pete confesses that he has already revealed his homosexuality first to his mother, since he knows, '"Dad can't stand the word 'gay,"' [...]. 'When he hears it, his face squishes up like a bird dropped something white out of itself down on Dad"'(90). He also adds, '"I never brought any women home. I never talked about any women. I'm twenty-seven years old"' (91). He acknowledges before Erick that Jim Stanley has inspired him to come out of the closet:

> "Jim's a political gay. I used to hate gay activists! I used to think they were a bunch of self-pitying sissies who blamed everything on the fact they were homosexuals. I used to tell Jim that what I did in bed was my own private business. Jim said that was right: What I did in bed *was,* but what about life out of bed? What about lying to everyone, trying to pass for straight, never letting family or friends know what was going on in my life?.... He convinced me the only way to get past that kind of self-hatred was to come out of hiding. He said anyone who loved me wouldn't love me any less if I came out, and I'd like myself a lot more. So I started with Mom. You were next on

> my list."(95)

Kerr here shows that the gay rights/liberation movement in the 1970s and 1980s in America following the Stonewall riot in 1969 in New York City's Greenwich Village has encouraged many gay people to come out of the closet. However, in the novel her emphasis is on covert homosexuality. This is indicated when she draws the analogy between Pete and the "night kites" that he himself makes and likes: "Pete said night kites are different, they don't think about the dark. They go up alone, on their own, Pete said. And they're not afraid to be different. Some people are different, too, Pete said" (12). This is further highlighted when Pete later says to Erick who is fond of conventional day kites, '"Oh, I'm a night kite'" (16). Here, Kerr draws a parallel between night kite and Pete, between the dark and the closet gayness. Perhaps she tries to explain the symbolic significance of the title of her novel. Again, she narrates a scene in which Pete admits that he has named his pet dog Oscar after the Irish writer Oscar Wilde (1854-1900) who was imprisoned for being a homosexual. Eric wants to know:

> [...], Oscar isn't named after Oscar *Wilde*, is he?"
>
> "That's who he's named after," Pete said.
>
> [...]
>
> "You were also probably the only one in the family who ever knew Oscar's last name," I said.
>
> "Or that he even had one," said Pete. (100)

Pete's homosexuality is objectified in the dog called Oscar. Through this equation of homosexuality with caninity, Kerr suggests that Pete's gayness is inconspicuous. She thus reinforces her preference for secret homosexuality that is once called 'the love that dare not speak its name' by Wilde's lover, Lord Alfred ("Bosie") Douglas. In so doing, she suggests that a homosexual is a deviant person, must not openly claim to be seen as a 'normal' human being. Another point is that Kerr reduces the status of human homosexuality to an animal state. In doing so, she ruthlessly marginalizes the gays, and provokes homophobia. Kerr seems to be a heterosexual bigot. In the history of the gay movement in the mid-1980s in America, closeted homosexuals were considered as the greatest obstacles to the homosexuals' progress, since they were seen as not having their integrity and as persons very useful to heterosexual establishment. Even their official or unofficial empowerment in various social and political spheres was seen as promoting anti-gay prejudices under which they chose to live because of their fear of coming into the open, of attracting stigmatization.

Pete's disclosure of his sexual orientation actually shocks his mother, even though just to please her son she says then, '"I wasn't *surprised.*'" and is rather glad '"Pete [...] wasn't a loner [...]'" (115). Erick takes it easy. He suggests to his mother, '"We shouldn't have a problem with his being gay, Mom"' (115). This is despite Erick being straight. His father who always talks to his two sons about sowing their wild oats, '"men and women and marriage'" and '"a lot of playing around'" (161) is brutally intolerant. He even cannot stand Erick having his arms around his best friend Jack. That is why, one day Eric angrily says to his mother, "[...] tell Dad not to worry, he has only one fag son, not two" (123). Kerr is comfortable to see Eric affirm his sexual identity, even as she loves to portray Pete keeping his gayness dark until he develops AIDS and thereby stresses that non-heterosexuals are pathological. She also shows her strong straight bias in her delineation of heterosexist father for whom homosexuality is acquired, abnormal and not natural: "'I'm not accusing anyone of anything! But maybe if we'd paid a little more attention to what Pete was doing when he was Erick's age, we wouldn't be in this situation!'"(134).

Pete however has failed to be in the open as gay,

which is why he frequently engages in unsafe sexual practices with multiple partners with the insatiable feeling of '"The more the merrier'"(179). He does not have any regrets about it:

> "Now I think about a lot of things I never thought about before. But I don't look back on my life and say I should have done this, or I shouldn't have done that, any more than anyone else dying probably does. You don't die at my age without regrets, or without thinking how you might have done things differently."(179)

Such is the positive attitude of HIV-positive Pete who has written an unfinished short story titled "The Sweet Perfume of Good-bye." The story is about the "world where there's no fragrance whatsoever until someone starts dying [...]" (215). Despite being tortured and crushed by the stigmatic gestures towards him, this spirit of endurance and acceptance sustains in Pete till the last line of the novel: "There's the sweetness first... and later on, the end" (216). These are the words of Pete. Kerr presents here what might be called "ego-syntonic homosexuality" (the condition of a person content with his or her homosexuality) that The American Psychiatric Association declassified as a mental illness in 1973.

When Pete's infection with HIV/AIDS is disclosed, everybody in the family refers to the disease as "a thing, a bug, everything but AIDS [...]" (98). The term AIDS is, as it were, a taboo word. Despite this, the father is very keen to take proper care of his son who has developed by then swollen lymph nodes and Kaposi's sarcoma. He brings Pete home. The novel then dwells on stigma and AIDS phobia. Mrs. Tompkins, their housekeeper tolerates Pete for sometime and then behaves differently towards him. She keeps Pete's dishes separately. Erick narrates, "And after that Mom found her doing Pete's sheets and pillowcases by hand in a tub filled with Tide and Clorox, [...] wearing rubber gloves.[...] she didn't think Pete's things should be laundered with everyone else's. It went on and on, and when Mom said we weren't going to live that way,[...] Mrs. Tomkins broke down and admitted that her daughter wanted her to quit, twenty years with us or not! Mrs. Tompkins was terrified, too" (173-74). She quits her job. No woman wants to work with them. Nicki Marr is dazed to hear that Pete has AIDS and breaks up her relationship with Erick. Her father even fears infection in the pool where Nicki and Erick have already swum together. He brainwashes her. On phone, Eric tries hard to convince her:

> "I don't have it, for God's sake!"
>
> "You could have it without knowing it, and give it to someone else. Daddy read that in a newspaper."
>
> "That's not true, Nicki. I can show you that in black and white!"
>
> "Maybe *I* could get it now."
>
> "*I* don't have it, Nicki! Pete has it, and I can't catch it from Pete! [...].
>
> [..]
>
> "Nicki?" I tried to keep my voice level. "I'd like to bring out a pamphlet about this thing. It explains that you can't get it from casual contact."
>
> "Casual contact," she said sarcastically.
>
> "*I* don't have it!"
>
> "Does that pamphlet explain why you didn't tell someone you supposedly loved that it's in your family?"
>
> "No," I said, "it doesn't explain that.... I'll try to explain that."

> "I don't see how you can," she said. [...]. (206-07)

Apparently, in this novel Kerr projects the homosexual as an aberrant individual and therefore an HIV-positive person. In fact, she effectively evokes HIV/AIDS as a gay disease. She finds it difficult to accept gayness as a valid sexual behaviour. It is rather for her a psychologically deviant behaviour. Coupled with this is the portrait of her phobic notion of homosexual AIDS. This reflects largely her heterosexual ideology that belongs to the hegemonic class.

Gloria D. Miklowitz in her novel *Good-bye Tomorrow* (1987) chooses the world of teenagers to treat the subject of HIV/AIDS. The novel deals with the mental anguish of an eighteen-year-old straight man who is infected through blood transfusion during his treatment in the wake of an accident that causes severe bleeding and fracture. He subsequently distances himself from his girlfriend to save her from being infected by him even as he experiences disgrace and disapproval in his family and school. Though the novel seeks to end on an optimistic note by making the HIV-positive young man socially acceptable, it fails to free itself from the homo-and-AIDS phobia that was rife in America in the 1980s. It thus supports the dominant perception of AIDS. It is obviously written from a straight perspective.

The Weiss family in Los Angeles includes Alex, his fifteen-year-old sister Christy, his father George and mother Beth. Alex is in the swimming team in school. He has plans to join college. Once he is seriously wounded in a car accident and is rushed to the hospital where he undergoes two blood transfusions. Within a year, he develops weight loss, night sweats, flu, lump in the throat and swollen lymph nodes. Observing the frequency of these symptoms, family physician Dr. Hoff recommends a blood test to check antibodies for the AIDS virus. The very mention of "AIDS" perplexes Alex:

> A cold sweat flushed over me. Gripping the arms of the chair, I leaned forward. "Did you say *AIDS*?"
>
> Hoff nodded, [...].
>
> "Why would you want to check me for that?" I blurted. "[...] I'm not *gay*!"
>
> "And you're not a drug user, either. I know that."
>
> "Then *why*?"
>
> "[...] you had a blood transfusion last year. Remember? I want to be sure you didn't pick up the AIDS virus from that transfusion."
>
> "Pick up AIDS through a single transfusion?"
>
> "*Transfusions*. You had two. It's not likely, but... yes. Last year, when you received those transfusions, there was no way to screen for the AIDS virus in a donor's blood. The reason I'm concerned is that we're seeing a lot of hemophiliacs who have tested positive. [...]."(56)

This conversation brings to the surface how Alex has internalized homophobia. It also draws the reader's attention to the common perception of HIV/AIDS as a "gay disease" in America in the 1980s. Miklowitz has no problem, no qualms in reiterating the hegemonic notion of the gayness of the disease in its early years. At a time when drastic intervention is needed to counter this dominant notion that costs thousands of gays their lives, she chooses to have the sadistic pleasure of writing the novel from the vantage point of heterosexuality. Alex gives his blood samples to Dr. Hoff for the ELISA test and then discovers himself in "a kind of trance, hands icy, mind numb" (58). Alex's major concern now is if he has infected his seventeen-year-old girlfriend Shannon Begley. He expresses his discomfiture thus:

> [...].I'd had two little transfusions. Hemophiliacs needed hundreds of donors' blood for one transfusion - no wonder they were at such risk. That made sense, didn't it?
>
> But what if I *did* get the AIDS virus through those transfusions? What if I did have HTLV-III?
>
> *I could have given it to Shannon!* AIDS was transmitted through sex as well as through blood or contaminated needles. Shannon and I had been intimate for most part of the year! If she caught the virus from me, then she was at risk for getting AIDS too!
>
> What should I do?
>
> [..]
>
> I pulled off the road onto a gravel shoulder, feeling as if *I* was rolling over the sharp stones, and turned off the engine. For a long time I just sat there [...] and cried. (58-59)

Alex's mental state suggests that the heterosexual transmission of HIV must be contained and that the straight community, projected as a 'normal' (and therefore 'healthy') population must be protected. Homosexuals, IV-drug users and hemophiliacs must be allowed to die of the disease. Miklowitz is quite comfortable in her homicidal way of looking at this devastating disease.

Withdrawn completely, Alex behaves like an introvert. In his friend circle any jokes concerning AIDS annoy him. He deliberately behaves very rudely towards Shannon to keep himself away from her. Shannon is stunned by the abrupt change in Alex's behaviour. So far Alex has not divulged his conversation with Dr. Hoff to anybody. He keeps waiting with terrible anxiety for the test result to come:

> [...]. I withdrew from everything- until I *knew*.

> And the knowing dragged on. I phoned Hoff's office every day to find out if the results of the ELISA were back, and every morning I woke up with my jaws aching from grinding my teeth. (68)

The test shows positive. However, for a hundred percent reliability Dr. Hoff gets Alex's blood drawn once again for Western Blot test with a consoling note, "Even if this does prove positive, it only means you've been exposed to the AIDS virus. It doesn't mean you'll *get* AIDS" (69). Hoff advises Alex to share his shock either with his parents or friends and wants to help him in this connection. However, Alex insists that his infection should not be disclosed. He then borrows books and clippings on HIV/AIDS from the school library, and, keeping himself locked in his room, reads them secretly again and again "with macabre intensity [...]"(70). However, the sudden change in his demeanour causes suspicion in Christy who succeeds in pressurizing Alex to unlock the door, darts into his room and picks up one of the AIDS articles. She then asks him, "[...]. All this change in you started right after you went to see the doctor. Did he say you had *AIDS*?" (72). Alex somehow manages to evade Christy's questions by saying that he is doing his school assignment. Christy checks with her boyfriend John (who is also the best friend of Alex) regarding her brother's school assignment, finds it to be a lie. She displays her affection for Alex, whereby she is able to learn from him about his infection with AIDS. She then panics, "[...], if Alex had it – could I get it? Could Mom and Dad?" (83).

In the hegemonic convention, HIV/AIDS is always depicted as something that is fearsome. Christy's fear gradually increases as she learns that the Western Blot test also shows positive: "I removed Alex's dishes—being careful not to lift the glass where his lips had touched—and pushed the cart out to the kitchen. I loaded the dishwasher, just as I always do, then, with the machine going so no one would hear, I turned on the water and washed my hands" (108). Alex observes their mother (Beth) responding disgracefully to his infection in presence of Dr. Hoff:

> "I'll see that Alex takes better care of himself," Mom said. "But what about the rest of our family? Christy? George and me? Is there any chance we could catch it?"
>
> "Beth!" Dad cried out, shocked. "Alex told you yesterday how it's contracted!"
>
> Mom made an apologetic hand gesture. "I know. I know. But can we get the virus if I launder his clothes with ours? If he uses the same utensils and glasses as we do? If one of us empties his wastebasket full of tissues when he's had a cold?"
>
> *She was afraid of me!*
>
> I couldn't bring myself to look at Mom. She should have waited to ask about that when I wasn't around! I shivered, aware for the first time that I was really alone in all this, that there was a wall between me and my family now. As much as they loved me, they were *afraid* of me. (92-93)

Here, the novelist presents irrational fear associated with the disease. She does not even spare a mother and a sister from being prey to unreasonable fear of an infected son and an HIV-positive brother and thereby, for a moment, sounds non-judgemental in her approach. At least she has chosen to sink or overlook the differences between "family" and "community" in so far as their stigmatizing responses to the HIV-positive people are concerned. Usually, in almost all HIV/AIDS narratives, "family" is projected as a last resort for the HIV-positive people. It is always shown as an idealized notion. Here, Miklowitz violates that convention. Of course, her depiction of phobic response to AIDS suggests that the disease terribly disrupts nuclear family ties, and deep emotional bonds as well.

Feeling stigmatized at home for sometime, Alex compulsively develops an obsession with the disease, "[...] everywhere I went I heard AIDS mentioned" (86). Alex's awareness of his own pathological complex is seen as he repeatedly explains to others, '"No. I've got the virus, but not the disease"' (127). It gets aggravated by the talk of the people around him. Afraid of being asked to quit swimming on grounds of his infection in school, at first he lies to his swim coach that he does not have AIDS. However, he reflects, '"But I can't live with a lie"' (131). He once again tells the coach, '"I don't have AIDS. I've got ARC"' (131). Its impact is that his swim mates do not want to bathe with him in the same pool. The coach tells him, '"[...]. They're scared that if you cut your foot and bleed on the locker-room floor and they walk on it, they'll get infected"' (131). The principal wants to suspend Alex from school, '"We just can't take chances with the health of our other students"' (136). He says, '"[...]. If you stay in school, there'll be objections from parents. Some people will take their children out of school. We have to consider all these things"' (136-37). This is in spite of Alex's entreaty, '"But I can't infect anyone! Not by just going to school!"' (137). Alex is extremely angry as he argues, '"It seems pretty hypocritical! I've had this infection for months, probably, not even knowing it. I didn't even have to tell anyone! I've been taking showers, swimming in the same pool, sharing the same drinking fountains all these months and you weren't worried then. Why now?"'(136). However, he is happy to learn that John in his absence has already argued strongly with the principal to convince him about the non-transmissible routes of HIV/AIDS. For a moment Alex regrets, "[...] Hoff was right—I shouldn't have admitted any thing. Look what being honest did. I was being suspended" (137). As his story hits the headlines of newspapers, he feels:

> As I read the story in the paper a cynical part of me thought, What a hell of a big fuss they're making over one high school kid! There had to be dozens of gay teachers, maybe even hundreds, teaching in the schools. Probably half of them carried AIDS antibodies. There had to be hemophiliacs going to school, who knows how many, who probably carried the virus too. And I bet there were more than a few druggies in each school who picked up the virus from infected needles. But I didn't hear all this hue and cry about them being a threat to others!
>
> Maybe I did good, after all, by admitting what I have. Now, my friends would have to take a stand. People would have to face up to the facts, instead of the imagined facts and fears about AIDS.
>
> Next week, when I went back to school, I would tell the tale. Would I still belong? Or had I become a nonperson? (143-44)

Though Alex has been portrayed as having the eagerness to fight, he does not demonstrate it actively and relentlessly. That is why, he seems to be a pathetic figure deserving of pity. Alex feels ostracized. His loneliness is further compounded by his sense of guilt, as he thinks of Shannon whom he believes to have infected. Alex consults Dr. Hoff who advises ELISA test for Shannon. After days of indifference, one day he meets Shannon who in turn feels helpless:

> He [...] blurted, "I have ... a virus... AIDS... not the disease, but the virus."
>
> "AIDS?!" I shivered. "I...I don't understand. It can't be!"
>
> [..]

"The worst of it is - I may have infected *you!*" he cried at last, in anguish. "It kills me to think that!"

[...]

"How?" I whispered. "We used precautions."

"Sure, so you wouldn't get pregnant. Not to prevent AIDS. Who would have thought you'd have been better off if we'd not switched to the pill."

[...].

[...]. "What do we do now?"

"We have to know. You have to go in for the ELISA test. Hoff expects you. I told him about us."

[...]

"Why?"

"Because if you contracted the virus from me, I couldn't live with myself! And if you haven't... then we have to stop going together."

[...]

"I couldn't stand not seeing you anymore! If it's sex you're worried about, we could just not do it! Or- you said there were safe ways...condoms."

"No."

[...]

[...]."What's going to happen to us? What do we do?"

"First, you're going to take the ELISA."

[...]

> [...]. I ached to run after him, to hold him, to tell him everything would be all right, to say I still loved him. But I didn't. (99-102)

Miklowitz is very effectively communicating the message of 'safe' teenage male-female sex in spite of and because of AIDS. She also presents successfully that heterosexual AIDS can also be harrowing. This is a redeeming feature of the novel. Shannon gets her blood tested by Dr Hoff. The first test shows negative. The doctor asks her to test again within two to three months, since after infection with HIV it takes anywhere from three weeks to six months for antibodies to develop. Shannon then instinctively reacts, "I started to shiver. At that moment, I hated Alex. None of the closeness we'd shared was worth this fear, this uncertainty, worth the chance I might have contracted the virus" (114). Of course, she feels shame later. However, Alex has resolved to save Shannon from being infected by completely breaking up their relationship and by abandoning her. He says to her: '"I'll never forget what we had, but it's over. It's good-bye tomorrow for me, at least that's how I see it. You gotta start seeing other guys..." (118).

This points to the justification of the novel's pessimistic title, though the story ends with a hopeful note. Shannon refuses to yield to Alex's pressurization not to see him anymore. Instead, she tries without his knowledge to persuade her friends to escort him into school. This is her confidence-building gesture. Her sole objective is to show to everyone that they are not afraid of an HIV-positive person. Initially she is desperate, since she does not get any friend to join her in her noble venture. Finally, she succeeds in persuading only one friend called Rob. The next day on his way to school, Alex is accompanied by Christy and John. He discovers that some students glance uneasily in his direction, while "[...] some guys passed as if nothing had changed, but I figured they just didn't know yet" (149). To all these,

John says to him, '"It's just your imagination'" (149). They are later joined by Shannon and Rob who exchange smiles with Alex, and five of them stroll "on through the parking lot [...] to school" (150). Despite AIDS, Alex has been treated rather as an 'insider' in a heterosexual community perhaps because he has been projected as an "innocent victim."

Alice Hoffman's *At Risk* (1988) is the story of an eleven-year-old white girl who contracts HIV through blood transfusion during her surgery for appendicitis and falls sick. It is mainly written from a heterosexual point of view. The novel touches the right chord in its readers primarily because the girl like any other child in any society is 'innocent' or culturally thought of as such. Moreover, Hoffman's skill in the use of rhetoric to depict vividly the plight of the child with AIDS and of her family that is consequently ostracized and stigmatized as well, in effect, also makes the story poignant. The novel apparently seeks to contest the phobic notion of HIV/AIDS by arousing in its readers sympathy for the girl and her family that are not to blame for the transfusion-related AIDS. Rather, it actually promotes the hegemonic construction of binary categories such as "the innocent" versus "the guilty,"and "the risk-groups" (obviously the homosexuals and the IV-drug users) versus "the general population" or "the heterosexuals." Ironically, the construction of these categories pertaining to AIDS was the prevailing cultural practice in America in the 1980s when the novel was written. Even in 1988, the year of publication of the novel, HIV/AIDS was regarded primarily as a gay disease. It is also appropriate to suggest that the novel also reminds its readers of real-life incidents involving hemophiliac schoolchildren like the three sons of Louise and Clifford Ray in Florida, Ryan White in Indiana and Mark Hoyle in Massachusetts who developed AIDS after transfusion, subsequently had to face, along with their families, severe death threats, social boycott, institutional discrimination and atrocities from the local American community of the 1980s.

The novel recounts the story of the Farrell family in Morrow, Massachusetts, a family that comprises Amanda, her eight-year-old brother Charlie, her father Ivan and her mother Polly. Ivan is an astronomer and teaches in a graduate institute, while Polly is a photographer with the spiritualist Laurel Smith and also an illustrator of some books written by the author Betsy Stafford. Stafford's son Sevrin is Charlie's best friend.

Amanda is devoted to gymnastics and proves herself to be one of the best gymnasts in elementary school. She has superb gym skill and competence. That is why her gym coach Jack Eagan, who also has a daughter named Jessie, admires her at heart: "There have been moments when he's wished that Amanda were his daughter instead of Jessie. Not that he doesn't love Jessie, he does, but Amanda is a champion. It's not just that she's good, it's that she wants to win. Badly" (107). Polly idealizes her daughter: "It still amazes Polly that this girl who can throw herself onto the uneven parallel bars with a grace that is almost like flight is her daughter. [...] When she watches her daughter compete, Polly feels [...], a piercing physical reaction to something extraordinary. At those times Amanda is not the child Polly covers at night with an extra quilt, the girl who leaves her leotards on the floor, [...] is a creature Polly cannot name, one made up not of flesh but of points of brilliant light"(16).

Hoffman creates a female character who is a figure of innocence together with uncommon sporting abilities. She projects Amanda as an unearthly person and idealizes the latter's innocence. Her strategy of portrayal of Amanda serves only to have a sentimentalizing effect on the readers.

One day immediately after scoring the highest points in a gymnasts' meet at school, Amanda vomits continuously and then develops fever. Gradually her knee joints swell. Her doctor Ed Reardon, who had earlier seen her through a worrisome appendectomy when she was given a transfusion, now does some blood and stool tests. Finally, Amanda tests positive for AIDS. Ed chooses to break this news first to "Ivan alone, without Polly," as Ivan being a scientist "could better accept the random path of a virus" (52). However, he is pretty sure that "No one can accept the indiscriminate order of cruelty" (53). Ivan's instant reaction zeroes in on those who have caused his daughter's illness. He makes Ed responsible for Amanda's sickness:

> [...]. It crosses his mind that he should kill Ed Reardon. Ed is the one who diagnosed Amanda's appendicitis. There was unexpected bleeding during her surgery; Ivan remembers being told she needed a transfusion. That was when she was given the contaminated blood. For five years Ivan has been losing her without knowing it. (54)

Ivan then blames the blood donors:

> [...].He has already told Polly that, as far as he's concerned, Amanda has been murdered. He is looking for suspects; if he could ever find out who donated the blood Amanda got, he could break that person's neck, he would listen to the bones snap. He'll never find that person, but from the way he was acting, it appeared that Ed Reardon was the next best thing. (58)

Here Hoffman shifts the focus away from Amanda to 'the others', who are projected as the diseased ones, are always seen as giving and spreading the illness. This is an issue that has been dealt with in Chapter-I. In this context, Ed and the blood donors (presumably homosexuals and IV-drug users with AIDS) are the 'others.' At another level, as Kruger rightly points out, "the novel moves closest to the distinction of 'guilty' and 'innocent' people with AIDS [...]" (128). The 'guilty' that appear unspecified in Ivan's imagination as "suspects" in causing the illness in 'innocent' Amanda is understood easily as HIV-infected gays and IV-drug users in dominant heterosexual mindset. By foregrounding this, the novel upholds the hegemonic ideology that does not subscribe to the rational notion that AIDS can infect anyone.

Perhaps as a saving grace, Hoffman introduces a minor HIV-positive character named Brian who "has been in love only with men, but [...] has slept with both men and women, and [...] shot cocaine [...], shared someone's needle" (138). He is a singer. Out of despair, Ivan regularly seeks telephonic counselling concerning Amanda's illness from Brian who "staffs the phone two nights a week" in an office of "an AIDS hotline in Boston, sponsored by a gay organization Ivan's never heard of" (100). He applies all types of therapeutic measures suggested by Brian to his daughter. It is Brian who suggests the name of a dentist who fulfils Amanda's last wish to take her braces off. This gesture comes at a moment when other dentists refuse to see her since she is HIV positive. Ivan depends emotionally and impulsively on Brian so much so that the former identifies his ailing daughter with the latter. In fact, Hoffman has hinted at this identification early in the novel when she talks about Jessie and Amanda who "are in love with some singer in a rock group, whom they refer to by his first name, Brian, as though they were on intimate terms with him"(29). Only once Brian is seen meeting Ivan. Otherwise he is portrayed as a telephonic voice, a disembodied 'noble' presence in the novel. Moreover, like Amanda, he does not die in the novel, even though both of them are indirectly presented in a death-like state. Apparently, the distinction between an 'innocent' Amanda and a 'guilty' Brian ceases to exist. However, as Katie Hogan in her article "Speculations on Women and AIDS" rightly argues, "[...] by rendering Brian as 'innocent' as Amanda, Hoffman sidesteps the more complex issue of the politics of the 'innocent victim' [...]"(88). In the same article,

Hogan also cogently questions the forging of alliance between Amanda and Brian "with a sentimental expression of sameness. Hoffman presents Brian, a bisexual man and former IV drug user and musician as both the composite of several 'outcast' identities on the one hand and then casts him as overwhelmingly acceptable on the other" (88). Another point to be noted is that heterosexuals turning to homosexuals for counselling despite homophobic perception of HIV/AIDS might seem as the erosion of boundaries between the two. However, the fact remains that in the 1980s, the latter being mostly affected by HIV/AIDS knew more about the disease than the former. They were the first to start many AIDS research organizations and help groups.

Contrary to Ivan's blame-attributing feeling towards Ed, Polly endorses her full faith in the doctor who subsequently sees HIV-positive Amanda through prolonged fever, weight loss, diarrhoea, and pneumonia: "She believes him. That is why Ed Reardon feels married to her. She believes him and only him, [...]" (156). Hoffman then juxtaposes the seriousness of Amanda's illness with Polly's apparent submission to adultery. Knowing for sure that Amanda would not survive, Ed always falsely assures Polly of her daughter's cure. Polly believes him. When Amanda has an attack of pneumonia, Ed speaks up to Polly: '"I can't lie to you anymore"' (161). He then takes Polly into his car, pulls her into his lap and she falls asleep in his arms. Both of them kiss and feel the sexual desire for each other. While sitting beside the sleeping Amanda in the hospital, "Polly can still feel the heat. It's so pure that when she leans down and kisses Amanda's forehead, the heat is transferred to her daughter, exactly where it belongs"(162). Kruger views this semi-romantic situation as a move towards "adultery" (129) and as the "breakdown of the nuclear family" (129) that HIV/AIDS has caused. He rightly argues, "AIDS leads not only to the isolation of the Farrell family from its community but to deep stress within the family itself, and AIDS is thus confirmed as a force deeply disruptive to the 'normal'" (129). However, Hogan looks at it from a different angle:

> [...] Hoffman clearly wants her readers to understand Polly's desire as irregular, as caused by the enormous stress and depletion associated with her child's dying from AIDS. The embrace and kiss are portrayed as warm, cuddly, affectionate, nonthreatening: it both unleashes and contains our culture's unconscious belief that AIDS is linked to every imaginable form of chaos—the demise of traditional families, the rise of non-monogamy, promiscuity and deviant sexual practices—while reassuring its readers that nothing of the sort will happen to them, even if one of their own should become ill and die. (89)

However, this sudden deviance in Polly who has been shown as living to serve the needs of the family may also be seen in the following light: 'heterosexual' desire or relationship, be it licit, monogamous, and familial or illicit, promiscuous, and non-procreative, is always already seen to be 'safe' from infection in spite of and because of AIDS, since it is a compulsory cultural norm. This points to the straight bias of the novel.

Ivan and Polly completely break down in tears. When they inform Amanda about her sickness, she gazes at them as though they have gone mad:

> "No, I'm not," Amanda had said, puzzled. "I'm not sick."
>
> While Ivan explained about the blood transfusion and the virus, Amanda chewed bubble gum and stared at the ceiling. When he was done, she sighed and said, "All right. How much school do I have to miss?"
>
> "We don't know about school," Ivan had said.

> [...]
>
> "I can't be sick!" Amanda screamed at them. "Don't you understand anything! I can't miss school!" (56-57)

When doctor Ellen Shapiro tries to explain to Amanda about her disease, she responds, '"I don't understand why kids get it'"(60). After sometime she says, "'I don't want to talk about this anymore,' [...]. 'I don't want to be here anymore'" (61). Hoffman makes Amanda a tragic figure arousing pity and fear in the readers.

The Farrell family is treated as the "accused" (92). Betsy Stafford panics when she learns about Amanda's infection. She feels perturbed thinking about her son Servin who always spends much of his time with Charlie. She says, '"[...]. They've shared lunches and God knows what else. [...] They may have shared the same bed"' (86). She does not even heed Laurel Smith's advice, '"You can't catch AIDS like a cold. You have to exchange blood or semen. You can't get it from any casual contact. Even if you live with that person, even if you're in the same family"' (86). She puts Servin in a different school and prevents him from meeting Charlie. When the members of the school board are notified of Amanda's illness, a meeting is called:

> The school board members ask Ed Reardon what will happen if Amanda cuts herself and bleeds on another child; they want to know if her saliva is dangerous. Not one of them is really listening when Ed explains that siblings of children with AIDS have shared toothbrushes and not come down with the virus. They don't hear him when he insists their children are more likely to be run down by a truck in their own backyard than to contract AIDS from Amanda. (92)

This hostility is followed by objections from several protesters calling themselves the Community Action

Coalition who want to keep Amanda out of school. This group distributes "fliers warning parents of the consequences of having an AIDS patient in a public elementary school" (95). Even Charlie is not spared from stigmatization. In the classroom no one wants to sit next to him. He therefore accuses his sister: "He'd like to strangle Amanda. He knows this is all her fault. She's the reason why everyone was staring at him, and he didn't even do anything; she's the sick one" (132).

Polly faces all humiliations apathetically: "She can no longer tell the difference between her anger and her sorrow. Her house might as well say CONTAMINATED on the front door. When she walks into a shop, even when she goes to the gas station to fill up the Blazer, people ignore her, people she's known for years, neighbors she used to have coffee with, shop owners who know her by name. If Amanda had cancer or a brain tumor, they'd be bringing her casseroles and cakes. They'd be filling up her gas tank for free" (190). Even Amanda's regular dentist Dr. Crosbie, like many of his counterparts, refuses to see her at a time when her only wish before death is to remove her braces. Amanda is barred from competing in a gymnastic event at school, since "[...] the parents of one of her teammates have a credible medical report that allows that there is a slight chance of infection to her teammates if her blisters bleed while she's on the uneven parallel bars and another girl with open blisters immediately follows her onto that piece of equipment" (147). At school Amanda overhears Mindy, her friend whispering audibly to another team-mate named Lori, '"Do you think she sat on one of the toilets? I'll never, ever use them again"' (123). Polly internalizes these responses centring on HIV/AIDS phobia and stigmatization so much so that when Charlie has a fever, she mistakes it for AIDS and gets into a fit as she keeps repeating '"He's got it"' (176). Here Hoffman depicts the social response to the Farrell family in the wake of Amanda's illness, and thereby succeeds in arousing sympathy. However, she does not intervene effectively in the cultural perception of AIDS. Only she performs, as it were, her routine duty to disseminate information about the disease through the school principal who either invites a group of doctors to speak to parents about HIV/AIDS or explains customarily to the students that AIDS can not be transmitted through a toilet or hugging. Some characters have been nice to Amanda out of sympathy again. For example, Amanda is scared of her gym coach Jack Eagan who is always in the habit of shouting. But after her illness, he speaks to her in a soft tone:

> "The thing is this," he says, uncomfortable, "if you're weak or you don't feel good, I don't want you to get hurt."
>
> "You must think I'm really stupid," Amanda says.
>
> [...]
>
> "I didn't say you were stupid," Jack Eagan says. [...] "You're a champion. Champions don't let themselves feel pain. That's why I'm worried."
>
> [...]
>
> "Are you just being nice to me because you feel sorry for me?" Amanda says hotly.
>
> "You know I'm not nice," Jack Eagan says. (107)

Jack's daughter Jessie who is Amanda's best friend tries to bolster the latter's morale:

> "I don't look sick, do I?" Amanda says.
>
> "You look great," Jessie says. "Your dress looks fantastic."
>
> Amanda smiles [...] until Jessie says, "If anyone says anything mean to you, I'll hit them."(103-04)

Is this Hoffman's intervention strategy? What can be done about the off-campus mentality of the same guardians, the same students and the people in general? How can it be persuaded or challenged? Where is the eagerness to understand and fight the phobic notion of the disease? Perhaps the novelist has chosen spiritualist Laurel Smith who is morbidly obsessed with death and spirit to do this job. Laurel, unlike others, visits Amanda frequently after the latter is diagnosed HIV positive. She affectionately brushes and braids Amanda's hair. Amanda also develops extreme liking for Laurel. She even spends one night in Laurel's house, even though their closeness is not tolerated by Polly who considers Laurel's presence ominous. In actuality, Laurel is excessively fond of HIV-positive Amanda without any motive. This is revealed when Amanda wants to know if Laurel can talk to her after her death:

> "Honey, I can't do that," Laurel says evenly.
>
> "Yes. You can." Amanda sits up and leans forward. "That's what you do. You're a medium."
>
> "They were dreams," Laurel says. She takes one of Amanda's hands in her own. "That's all they were."
>
> Amanda pulls her hand away and studies Laurel. "Maybe you could. You could if you really wanted to."
>
> [..]
>
> "No," Laurel says. "Not even if I really want to."
>
> "I thought you'd be able to talk to me," Amanda whispers. (180)

At least Laurel has honest care for Amanda. The behaviour of the schoolchildren terribly hurts, upsets Amanda and fills her with self-hatred, with an intense feeling of the certainty of her death from the disease:

> [...]. They hate her, she knows. She doesn't even blame them; she hates herself too, not all of her, just this thing that's inside her. At first, she didn't really believe it because when she looked at herself in the mirror, she looked exactly the same, just thinner. She used to tell herself all she had to do was wait and they'd find some shot or pill they could give her. Now, every night before she goes to sleep she tells herself that she's going to die. She repeats it to herself, calmly, carefully, rolling the words on her tongue. (123)

She also demonstrates this feeling at home when over the dinner at the table she angrily argues with her parents who do not allow her to attend a birthday party and have a sleepover:

> "You hate me," Amanda says to her parents.
>
> She has a terrible look on her face. She pushes the plate of cake away from her, hard. The plate skitters across the table and crashes on the floor.
>
> "We love you," Polly says. [...]
>
> "Oh, yeah," Amanda says. "Sure. That's what you say. You have to say that."
>
> "This is not up for discussion," Ivan says. "You can go to the party, but you can't sleep over."
>
> "Just embarrass me in front of everybody," Amanda cries. "My life is ruined anyway."
>
> Her words fall across the table like splinters of glass. They should be eating chocolate cake, instead they are bleeding from their souls. [...] Amanda glares at her parents, defying them to try to comfort her.
>
> "Amanda," Polly says. "Please."
>
> "Please what?" Amanda fires back. "Please just

> die and get it over with?"
>
> [..]
>
> Nobody tries to stop Amanda as she runs outside. [...] Amanda [...] starts to cry. Stupid, but it was only at the dinner table that she realized in order to die of a disease you really have to die and not come back. (115-17)

Despite all these agonies, Amanda's love for sports continues. In order to participate in a gym meet, she argues before her coach Jack, "'I'm not that sick!'[...]. 'I don't even look sick!'"(148). She becomes the winner in the gym meet and is congratulated by all. When invited by Jessie for dinner, she refuses and says to her, "'I won't be around forever,' [...]. 'You've got to start making other friends now'" (152). Finally, as Amanda is taken to hospital, she wills her possessions such as jewellery, art folder, cassettes and cassette player and gym bag to Jessie, her grand parents, Laurel and Charlie respectively. To her parents she bequeaths "everything else" (215). In the novel, she is last seen waving her hand that moves "like a piece of white paper" (215).

The novel promotes opposition between the guilty and the innocent. Despite its depiction of stigmatization due to infection with HIV/AIDS, this classification of HIV- positive identity strikes the readers.

Penny Raife Durant's novel *When Heroes Die* (1992) deals with the illness and subsequent death of a young gay man, whose charming personality and success as sportsperson makes the loss all the more sorrowful. It is written from the perspective of his nephew, a twelve-year-old boy, who watches his uncle die a shameful, agonizing death. As Gary Boyden discovers his uncle's diseased homosexuality, he also discovers his own 'normal' heterosexual desire in growing up, a desire that he finds complex and traumatic. Though it appears sympathetic to gay men's plight in the epidemic, the novel actually reinforces homophobic ideas even as it seeks to dispel them.

Gary's uncle Rob Lewis was a "star basketball player" for his school and university (132), and had won many trophies for his excellence. Clearly, the allusion is to Magic Johnson, basketball star turned HIV-positive campaigner for AIDS awareness, who is even mentioned in the novel (111). Johnson was lead player of the Los Angeles team Lakers, winning for them five National Basketball Association championships and later captained the U.S. Olympic team. He tested positive in 1991, after which he resigned from the game and counselled HIV-positive teenagers, for whom he was a role model.

A handsome and well-behaved young man, Rob is liked by everyone even after they learn of his homosexuality and of his death from AIDS:

> Gary was surprised by the number of people who brought food to their house and came to the funeral. People had always liked Rob, Gary knew that, but he thought that they might shy away because he'd had AIDS. He'd been wrong. People mourned for Rob all the same. (118)

Gary is deeply fond of his uncle and admires him. His father deserted his mother Wanda when he was still an infant, and her brother Rob has been their only support. For Gary, Rob is like a surrogate father: "Rob had caught him whenever Gary had started to fall. As long as Rob was around, Gary felt safe. Taken care of. Like Rob was his guardian angel. A father" (14). He teaches Gary how to play basketball, how to be 'cool' and date girls and how to grow up, and Gary looks upon his uncle as a "role model" (71).

One day while playing basketball Gary discovers that his uncle is seriously ill and has been ailing for some time. His mother tells him that Rob has AIDS, but he refuses to believe it and assumes instead that the blood report is wrong. Gary finds it deeply disheartening to accept his uncle's disease and prefers to deny it to himself and to others. But he is gradually persuaded of the truth by his mother and by Christie, the girl who lives next door. Christie's mother Mrs. Gilbert is a nurse and knows about Rob's illness.

The novel presents two simultaneous lines of action, both centered around Gary. The first concerns Gary's discovery of his uncle's illness and his sexual orientation, his initial shock and denial, and his eventual acceptance as he watches Rob die. The other deals with Gary's love affair with Shanna Wright, a girl who studies with him in Tyler Middle School. The story shifts back and forth between Rob's illness and Gary's pursuit of Shanna, a pursuit that is aided by Rob's advice and encouragement. The juxtaposition of homo and heterosexuality is necessary to guide Gary into a 'normal' adulthood, and it is significant that Rob provides this guidance.

When he first learns of his uncle's illness, Gary's reaction, as already stated, is a mixture of shock and denial: "Maybe it was a mistake. Maybe they had messed up in the lab and had the wrong person" (15). Later, when Christie and Wanda convince him that Rob is indeed HIV positive, he wonders how he could have got infected. He has not taken a blood transfusion, is not an IV-drug user and does not appear to be a homosexual. When his mother tells him that Rob is gay, he finds it even more difficult to accept and feels betrayed. The knowledge of Rob's sexuality triggers off a crisis, and Gary begins to fear that he may be gay too. He is also terrified of other's reactions, and tries to keep his uncle's disease a secret. The stigma of homosexual AIDS troubles him deeply, and he does not even want to think about it.

Meanwhile, Rob's pneumonia gets worse and he has to be hospitalized. Gary visits him in the hospital and is shocked to see him so ill. He visits him again and takes him out into the hospital's courtyard on a wheelchair. The two visits help Gary accept the reality of his uncle's disease and sexual orientation and strengthen the bond between them. Despite the shock he has received, his love and admiration for Rob remain the same. Soon after Gary leaves the hospital, Rob's condition turns serious suddenly, and he dies. It is only after his death that Gary learns how much people love and adore Rob, and that knowledge of his illness and homosexuality has not made any difference to their adoration. Rob wills his new car to his sister and his basketball trophies to his nephew. The novel ends with Gary's fond memories of the uncle he loves and admires, despite the fact that he was a homosexual who died of AIDS. Gary's final tribute to Rob's memory is his decision to play basketball again, which he had given up since the day he learnt of his uncle's illness, and to become like his uncle a star player.

Thus, Durant presents Rob's story not directly, as an account of what he underwent, but indirectly through the reactions of Gary. The focus on Gary achieves two things. First, Durant is able to present the story of homosexual AIDS without running the risk of forcing her readers, who are presumably straight, to identify with what is commonly perceived as a deviant sexuality. It is not Rob's trauma that is at the centre of the story but Gary's, thereby making it easier for the reader to empathize with the boy's loss rather than his uncle's agony. By thus displacing the trauma, Durant is able to forestall homophobic responses to Rob's death even as she presents homosexuality as abnormal. Secondly, by focusing on a child's suffering she is able to elicit greater sympathy, in much the same manner that children with AIDS appear more deserving of our pity than adults. Gary may not be an 'innocent' child 'victim' of AIDS, but an 'innocent victim' of the *tragedy* of AIDS he certainly is.

It is interesting to see how Durant handles the problem of homosexuality and the resurgence of homophobia in the AIDS epidemic. In the 1970s in America, after Stonewall and the gay rights movement, homosexuality had been decriminalized and had been taken out of the American

Psychiatric Association's list of classified mental illnesses. With the emergence of AIDS it was once again seen as pathological, though not officially so, as doctors tried to argue that AIDS was a 'gay disease.' In the mid-1980s the number of heterosexual cases increased significantly, Magic Johnson's being a well-known instance, but the stigmatization of gay sexuality continued. Durant's novel is presumably an attempt to fight this stigma and to persuade its readers that it is wrong to discriminate against gays.

The novel tries to foster sympathy for gay people by presenting an HIV-positive gay man who is liked and respected by all. The message is that one may be gay, but not therefore necessarily bad. When Wanda reveals to her son that Rob is gay, she tells him: '"Being gay doesn't make him a bad person, Gary. Some people think so, but it doesn't. He's still your uncle, and he's been a good uncle to you for years. Nothing can change that'" (70). When Gary tells Christie about his uncle's sexual orientation, she replies: '"It doesn't change what a great guy he is'" (84). Even his friend Sam, who strongly dislikes "fags" and openly expresses it, thinks that Rob '"was still a great guy to have for an uncle'" (124). Rob's funeral is attended by many of their friends and neighbours, who do not shun them, as Gary had feared, but rally round them in their grief. At school, Gary finds to his surprise that his teachers and friends are extremely supportive, and even those who hardly know him try to comfort him: "Some of the kids came up to Gary and said they were sorry. Others who had never noticed him before smiled at him in the halls. It made Gary uncomfortable to have attention focused on him. He hadn't done anything to deserve it" (120). However well-intentioned Durant's attempts at 'explaining' homosexuality may be, one thing is clear: what she ends up emphasizing is not the acceptability of homosexual desire but the large-heartedness of heterosexuals who do not bear their deviant fellow beings any grudge. This idyllic picture of a small- town American community that has overcome its homophobia is only too good to be true. The novel completely glosses over the reality of hate attacks and the government's criminal negligence of the plight of gay men in the early years of the epidemic.

The only homophobic character in the novel seems to be, ironically enough, Gary himself. Despite his great love for Rob, he cannot bring himself easily to accept his gayness:

> Why hadn't Rob told him the truth? Gary felt foolish, betrayed. Probably everybody knew. But not Gay. *He'd* thought his uncle was absolutely perfect!
>
> He turned over in his bed and pummeled his pillow with his fist. How could Rob have done this? His whole life was a lie! He had been Gary's hero, his role model. Some role model - getting himself sick, dying from AIDS.
>
> He had imagined scenes starring his uncle with all the beautiful women who were attracted to him. But Gary couldn't imagine the same scenes with his uncle and another man.
>
> Gary buried his head under the pillow, trying to blot out all the mental images of Rob. His stomach churned over and over again. *Why didn't he tell me? Why? Why?* (71)

The novel recounts Gary's transformation from homophobia to an understanding of gay people like his uncle. At first, his hatred of homosexuality manifests itself as a fear of being gay himself, of having inherited it from his uncle: "Was homosexuality inherited? If he was a 'real guy' wouldn't he have told Shanna to call? Wouldn't he have known how to handle it? A straight guy wouldn't just run from the girl of his dreams, would he?" (77). When Sam jokingly accuses him of being gay because he is too shy to talk to Shanna, he turns almost into a paranoid. His mother tells him that he is a lot like his uncle, good and kind and with a great sense of humour. However, Gary is too conscious of the fact that Rob was different, that he "was gay." Wanda explains to him that that was only '"a part of Rob. [...] it wasn't a part that made any difference in your life with him'" (134). In the final scene of the novel, Gary becomes Rob minus his gayness as he tries to relive his memory of his uncle and to identify with him.

Wanda's words to Gary on two occasions reveal an ambiguity that underlies her view of homosexuality, however sympathetic it may be. In the first, the context is the property that Rob bequeaths to his nephew, both literally and metaphorically. '"You'll always have parts of Rob,'" she tells her son after Rob's death, '"because he was with you while you were growing up. [...] But I hope you'll learn to be a parent, even without a father around'" (134). In other words, she wants Gary to be like Rob *minus* his problematic sexuality, to be what Rob could never have become, parent. The allusion here is also to her former husband, who fathered a child but refused to be its "parent." It is not simply heterosexuality that she wishes for her son, but a responsible and monogamously reproductive heterosexuality that both his uncle and his father lacked. If Wanda does not blame homosexuals, she does not think of them as 'normal' either. The second occasion is when she reveals to Gary that Rob was gay. '"I wish he weren't gay,'" she muses, '"*because he probably wouldn't be sick now,* and he deserves a longer life. But we can only guess what his life would be like if he were straight'" (70, italics added). The assumption here is that only gay people get AIDS, which was quite a false assumption to hold in the early 1990s. By then it had been established beyond doubt that AIDS was *not* a 'gay disease,' and there is even a reference to this fact in the novel. The book on AIDS that Christie gives to Gary states that "while most of those with sexually transmitted AIDS were gay, heterosexuals were beginning to test positive for the disease as well" (69). It is not Rob's gayness but his failure to practise safe sex that leads to his infection. To assume that Rob is sick *because* he is gay, therefore, is to be typically heterosexist and homophobic - underlying it is the idea that gay sexuality is diseased and that the gay man is *always already* infected even before the virus has entered his bloodstream. Homosexuality, therefore, is to blame for AIDS even as Wanda argues that gay men should not be blamed. Wanda Boyden is neither a minor character in the novel, nor are her statements presented with irony. It is she who is primarily responsible for the change in Gary's attitude, and her views are central to the novel's constructions of AIDS and homosexuality. The ambiguity underlying her views, therefore, reveals a latent homophobia in Durant's seemingly spirited defence of the gay community.

It is significant in this context that Durant does not represent the gay community, but a lone gay individual in a community that is comprised totally of heterosexuals. There is no mention of any gay lover who attends his funeral or visits him in the hospital or at home. By presenting Rob thus, the novel distances him from his troubling sexuality so that he is gay but not obviously so. Rob's homosexuality is sanitized and made acceptable by keeping it invisible, and by presenting it as a condition that he has no control over. '"Scientists now think that a person's sexual orientation is determined before he's born,"' Wanda explains to her son. '"It isn't something you choose. It's something you are"' (70). Rob is therefore not responsible for his homosexuality and cannot be blamed for it. However, there is something quite disturbing about this argument: if homosexuals cannot be blamed because they *have not chosen* their sexuality, it only follows that they can be blamed if they *have*. In other words, Wanda's argument does not counter the homophobic accusation but only side-steps it.

The threat of homosexuality is contained in the novel

by presenting Rob in a family setting, thus divesting him of his deviance. The 'good' homosexual is the one who never displays his homosexuality, who atones for his sin by being a supportive brother, an ideal uncle, a courteous neighbour and a committed citizen who supports "the local AIDS research project at the university" (119). Homosexuality is perceived as a threat to the family; therefore Rob must be shown as devoted to his sister's family, in contrast to Wanda's husband who deserts it. The novel repeatedly shows how deeply Gary trusts and depends on his uncle, who fulfils the responsibilities that his father did not: "He'd dreamed that Rob was his real father, not that other man whose picture was in the photograph album. Not the creep who ran out on them when Gary was only a baby" (78). In depicting Rob as an idealized 'good' homosexual, Durant does not counter the homophobic stereotype of the 'bad' homosexual but merely confirms the binarism.

Rob's death is his final atonement for the sin of his sexuality: "Gary went in for one last goodbye. So little of his uncle was left beneath the covers. AIDS had worn away his muscles, faded his tan, and finally, taken his breath. Death had replaced the panic breathing with a peaceful half smile" (118). He can now bequeath to his nephew his good "parts," his "trophies," while his bad "part" can be laid to rest forever. After the trauma of discovering his uncle's secret life, Gary can be reconciled to Rob only through the latter's death, which erases, as it were, his homosexual past. The melodramatic plot of *When Heroes Die* functions like the 'human interest' stories in newsmagazine accounts of the epidemic which, as Yingling notes, "are constructed to ensure an emotional response as the only certain response to an irresolvable social problem that calls forth numerous other *un*certain responses" (21).

4

Counter-hegemonic American HIV/AIDS Fiction

As has already been discussed in the introductory part of the preceding chapter, the counter-hegemonic practice in HIV/AIDS fiction seeks to demonstrate assertion of identity threatened with erasure and thereby resists the convention of projecting HIV-positive people as "non-beings." Its activist mode aims at securing the meaningfulness of HIV-positive life and in doing so allows, to quote Yingling, "an affirmation of identity not fated to succumb to the traps of affirmative, bourgeois culture in its determination to seal that identity and those meanings in a world of alienation and death" (54). Counter-hegemonic disease-discourse critiques the dominant constructions and seeks to represent the existence or authentication of selfhood by affirming it. Usually the off-family location is chosen as the platform to perform it through melodramatic, romantic or ironic modes. To demonstrate this viewpoint on the disease, the novels chosen are Paul Monette's *Afterlife* (1990), Vance Bourjaily's *Old Soldier* (1990), Christopher Davis's *Philadelphia* (1993) and Charlotte Watson Sherman's *Touch* (1995).

Paul Monette's *Afterlife* (1990) is about life after HIV/

AIDS. It deals with how three HIV-positive gay men live after the death of their AIDS-infected lovers. Its message is that HIV-positive persons should be able to reconcile themselves to their past, and always live in the present while continuously fighting the disease with the awareness of their future limitations. The novel has three plots, which despite their sudden twists and turns are interwoven into each other. It is written from a homosexual perspective even though it clearly targets heterosexuals. The way Monette depicts his gay characters in his novel makes his readers feel that as though he is living in an 'always-already' gay world. Just as heterosexuality is taken for granted, similarly for Monette, it seems, homosexuality is a natural given and not a historical construct. He uses heterosexually understood vocabulary to give expression to gay relationship. In so doing, he deliberately collapses the social structures of sexual categories. As with his biography *Borrowed Time: An AIDS Memoir,* in this novel Monette himself being gay and infected with AIDS celebrates gay and HIV-positive identities in an exuberant manner. The novel thus is about what might be called, to use his phrase in the novel, "dating in the apocalypse" (89). Monette deals with his subject through telling the life stories of three HIV-positive gay men who live in Los Angeles. Steven Shaw, Dell Espinoza and Sonny Cevathas come to know about one another at Cedar-Sinai hospital in Los Angeles where their three gay lovers are hospitalized and subsequently die of AIDS in the same week. They have been mourning the death of their lovers every Saturday night at Steven's house for one year. This is their "Saturday widowers' gatherings" (5). As the novel progresses, Monette weaves the three plots of Steven's growing love for Mark Inman, Dell's uncontrollable anger resulting in his act of terrorism, vandalism, killing and suicide, and Sonny's reckless sexual practices coupled with his inquiry into the New Age into a single narrative.

Steven is the central figure, and others rotate round

him. He has "the housemother instinct" and hence, to all other characters, has "simply been a sanctuary [...]" (275). In fact, his house has been the location for the convergence of all plots and all other characters. Sonny and Dell subsequently come to stay with him. Steven runs a travel agency called Shaw Travel. Following the death of Victor Diamond, his HIV-positive lover for eight years, grief-stricken Steven becomes a masochist. For fear of being "left with nothing" (2), he does not like to part with Victor's things. His distress prevents him from doing his work at his office: "He didn't want to hear about anyone going anywhere, which was why he stayed out of the office. Shaw Travel mocked him now [...]. For Steven travel was over. He'd become a walking bad advertisement, like a misspelled sandwich board" (9). He has even forgotten to love once again, "[...] he hadn't looked in anybody's eyes in over a year, not since the light began to go for Victor. Not even in his own eyes, not even in the mirror" (18). He refuses to have any pleasure or desire. He therefore has avoided all movies, malls and public events. "The only groups Steven ever saw anymore were at funerals" (71). Lovelorn Steven's melancholia and introversion evoke more of heterosexually perceived romance tradition than of tragedy. In so doing, Monette sidetracks the issue of tragedy and threat that HIV/AIDS poses. Readers are rather invited to watch an HIV-positive gay man who is pining away from romantic love.

However, Steven's obsession with despondency begins to change when in their Saturday evening's funeral he meets Mark Inman, television actor-producer and chief executive officer of a company. Mark tells Steven that he is HIV positive and that he had also been Victor's lover some ten years ago, as both of them look at Victor's pictures in Steven's photo albums. This revelation helps Steven connect to Mark and revive interest in love again. This feeling then was in his subconscious mind. For a moment, Steven tries to be intimate and expects Mark to cry for the loss of their friends to AIDS. However, Mark remains indifferent, "'I can't cry,' Mark announced [...]. At that he withdrew his hand from Steven's touch, restoring the equal distance, man to man [...]" (17). Even as Mark is not attracted to Steven, Steven develops love for the former, gets hurt in the process. He becomes lovesick. Despite this, one day Steven succeeds in experiencing his first date with Mark in a restaurant where both of them enter into an argument over their HIV-positive status. Mark feels uncomfortable to accept his infection and insists that he would commit suicide to avert the horrifying destruction of his body that AIDS would cause: "'Soon as I get sick, I'm checking out'" (66). Steven however responds with optimism, "'You don't know that, [...]. You'll probably want to fight for a while, and besides, the drugs might keep us going. Five years, maybe ten'" (66). After sometime he adds, "'Well, [...] sometimes people stick around for other reasons. So they can stay with people they love'" (67). Conventionally, all HIV-positive characters never wish to see the body disfigurements of their friends, since blemishes remind them of their own coming plight. Monette shows this in the character of Mark and at the same time counters the notion of the perishing HIV-positive body. In so doing, he advocates that despite AIDS one can continue to live and love life.

Day by day, Mark becomes an erotic catalyst for change in Steven, who gradually moves from "the fugue state of desirelessness" (152) caused by Victor's death to the revival of interest in sex. He is reborn sexually. He manages to have his first non-penetrative sexual involvement with Mark who is somewhat detached in bed, "'Don't you think we'll make better friends than lovers?'"(86). Steven subsequently engages himself in manual stimulation of sex: "Meanwhile, the only notable change in his own dysfunction was a most ambiguous gift of heat. Now he jerked himself off [...] every night [...]. But the fantasies were very careful – never Mark, certainly never Victor. In fact, he found himself roaming way back, to [...] dicks of the ancient world. The deep past was the one safe place where a man could still let go" (152). Monette obviously refers here to the gay unconscious, which is believed by all homosexuals to have been derived from ancestral memory or experience and thereby reinforces the historicity of gay identity that goes past the Stonewall riot in 1969 and subsequent gay rights movement in America in the 1970s to the ancient Greek society, where, as Foucault has shown in his *The History of Sexuality,* the same-sex desires, pleasures and social bondings were regarded as natural and sacred. The terms such as "marriage" and "wife" were introduced only in transition from ancient Greece to ancient Rome during the first two centuries AD. "Heterosexuality" since then has been seen as the "natural" and compulsory norm in direct opposition to 'homosexuality" that has been denaturalized, and associated with fear and hatred known as "homophobia." Monette is referring to this historical situation.

Steven continues to develop his love for Mark, who is more interested in friendship than in love. Monette then creates a patriarchal, heterosexual family to encourage male bonding and homosexuality. Mark confesses his HIV-positive status and his disinterestedness in Steven to his father Rob who has married a woman named Roz following the death of his first wife. He is surprised to hear the extolment of glory of love from his heterosexual father who encourages his son not to sever closeness, "'That's all there is, son. Someone to love. [...] The lucky ones are like Roz and me, we get another chance. We know it's not for long. [...] But it's all there is, so you'll take even a little. Everything else is shit"' (178). This advice brings about a transformation in Mark who afterward changes his repulsive attitude to his own HIV-positive status, gets intensely attached to Steven: "They were laughing now, giddy from so many feints, duelists sick of honor. They grappled into a breathless embrace, holding each other steady. And Steven made his final demand, swearing it like a blood oath: 'You can't die, okay? Not for years and years. I won't go through it again"' (232). Their sexual love demands its promise of perpetuation in the face of uncertainty. Eventually, their involvement also helps overcome Mark's reluctance to accept his HIV- positive status. Mark then quits his job with his boss Lou Ciotta, who was filled with pity and fear the moment the former told the latter about his infection with AIDS, '"[...]. Well, he pushed his chair back a couple of feet, and he stared at my teacup. [...] he was trying to figure out what I'd touched in the house"' (121).

Gradually both Steven and Mark learn to cope with HIV/AIDS. For example, at the funeral of Ray Lee, his employee at Shaw travel who is gay and dies of AIDS, Steven is restless and wants to leave. Monette writes, "Steven wasn't thinking of Ray or even Victor. He held himself back, abstracted, almost bored, yet hungry to be out of here and back in the soup of life. He felt selfish and loved the feeling, greedy to have his time with Mark" (259). With the new lover Mark, Steven wants to do away with his past symbolized by Victor and refuses to meditate on what is foretold for him by the death of Ray. Towards the end of the novel, Steven and Mark are alone together in bed in the former's house. Their friend Sonny is leaving Steven's house permanently. Another friend Dell has already left his (Steven's) house and killed Mother Evangeline and himself in the church. These things happen on the same morning. Dell's sister Linda rings Steven up to help her claim her brother's body. In these shocking situations, all Steven wants to do is to go back to bed even as he promises Linda over phone he would be right over there:

> He hung up the phone and swam back to the bedroom, a man whose privacy had been restored at last, [...]. Mark was still lying on his back, arms

> across his face. [...] Steven [...] crawled into bed beside the man he was still too shy to call his lover, [...].
>
> [...]. Mark stirred and reached an arm about Steven's neck, holding him tight [...]. Still half in a dream, he murmured: "What was all that?"
>
> "Nothing," Steven whispered. "Just the tenants leaving."
>
> Mark accepted the half-truth unquestioningly, [...] and burrowed into a full embrace. He felt the swell of Steven between them and mumbled, "You horny?"
>
> "Uh-uh-let's just sleep," replied his friend, swooning now in the warmth of the body that held him, letting go of all his fellow widowers. Even going under he could taste the simple wish that over-rided all the rest: to stay in the middle of this with Mark as long as he could. Perfectly selfish, except it was deeper than that - the last dance, the last pocket of air. Nothing else was happening right now in Steven's house, a luxury beyond calculation. The sleepers had all they needed. Only to lie like this between the bombs, dreaming away and not alone, because time was very short. (277-78)

Through Steven, Monette elicits a resisting response ("to stay in the middle of this") to the HIV-positive status in spite of the death threats ("the bombs") the disease poses. For Monette, to have lived and loved intensely despite being infected with AIDS is enough and is the most important way to hold the identity of the infected high.

In contrast to Steven, who accepts his infection and decides to live life only in the present, Dell Espinoza has a killer's instinct, and always broods over the past associated with his lover Marcus Flynn, the professor of

Mayan anthropology who died from AIDS. Dell is a gardener. Both of them met on a highway. "Bumper-to-bumper traffic, southbound on the 405 - Marcus in lane 2, Dell in lane 3, flirting like truckers all the way to Laguna. How else did professors and gardeners meet?"(57). This is in fact a rhetorical question signifying that gay love is not at all different from straight love and does not consider class. Monette parallels homosexuality with heterosexuality and wants his readers to see this. Dell and Marcus are HIV positive. However, Dell's sister Linda and Marcus "were captivated by each other" (53). Moreover, Dell suspects that Linda is a dyke when he sees her with her friend Emilia. Ironically, he is not happy about it as he says to Marcus, '"I just don't want some fat-ass dyke puttin' the moves on my little sister" (55). Himself being a queer, he cannot tolerate the idea of lesbianism. Marcus rebukes and calls him "sexist stereotype" (55). Monette here draws attention to the feminist's argument for female's distinct identity. Dell then suggests to Marcus to marry his sister. Therefore, at a much later stage Dell succeeds in getting Marcus (who was then wheelchair borne following his debilitation from full-blown AIDS) married to Linda. After Marcus's death, Dell and Linda become widows and are unable to overcome grief. Particularly Dell is consumed by the thought of his lover, "Almost unconsciously, not moving his lips, he prayed his double prayer. First to God, if there was a God, that He should reunite Dell and Marcus Flynn in heaven. [...] The second prayer was to Marcus himself, that he should protect his widows" (52).

Being unable to get a partner to replace Marcus, Dell remains sexually starved. He tries sex on phone. This is reminiscent of telephone sex that was practised as prophylactic apparatus during the AIDS epidemic in America in the 1980s when the novel was written. To all his calls, the response from the listener is "Someday" (51):

> [...]. In the country of 976, meeting was like commitment, a marriage doomed from the start. *Someday* meant no. Reality would only spoil it. Face to face they would see that one was still in high school, the other one old enough to be his father. Then what fantasy would they play?
>
> Yet both of them knew they would speak again. Dell never said a word about himself, or anyway not the truth, especially that Marcus had died of AIDS. In a jerkoff scene it was very bad form to bring up one's lover, let alone the holocaust. Dell was content to be a kind of scoutmaster to his 976 screw. When he called around he changed like a chameleon- sometimes Italian, sometimes twenty-five, top with bottom urges, rapist, virgin - anything not to be one particular man, especially himself.
>
> [...]. His hundred men with their vital stats were too familiar, too predictable, as hard to quicken as a sleepy wife. Of course he could go back into the pile, pay his twenty cents a minute to the LOAD line and start a new page. But he already had one of every kind. (51-52)

Through Dell, Monette is attacking the practice of telephone sex that aims at bringing sexual fantasy and reality together. Insatiability of sex over phone and impossibility of replacement of Marcus by someone else as lover fill Dell with rage. Dell rails at AIDS and even at God:

> Between God and Marcus he could only believe in one at a time, and Marcus always won. God was back in Morelia, the queer priest in his gold cloak seething for the altar boys, Beatriz and her useless novenas. God didn't have enough rage. No doubt the pederast Fathers of Morelia would

> have found it remarkable that Dell was praying at all. [...]
>
> But Dell was much further gone than that. He believed the opposite of everything, now that the anger had gone underground. [...] Not even revenge was enough of a reason to believe, for he couldn't pin the enemy down to any one man. Chaos was what mattered. Watching the world unstring itself, with just a snip of the thread here and there.
>
> Not that he wished to hurt anyone, except maybe God Himself. [...]. To go forward at all anymore, it wasn't a matter of faith but will. [...] Every single night before he went to sleep, he had to be finished with the world, in case he woke up too sick to go on. All he knew was this: before he went he would do what he had to, whatever it was, to let them know his people wouldn't go quietly anymore. (52-53)

This is the portrait of an angry young HIV-positive gay man. Through Dell, Monette wants his readers to remember historical figures such as Larry Kramer the dramatist who had shown in his writings his fury against the heterosexual bigots almost in a similar vein. In his relentless quest for more "chaos," Dell virtually turns out to be a rebel, a hotheaded vandal and an AIDS terrorist. His chaotic mental state is without any method and as complex and incomprehensible as AIDS itself. For example, he terrorizes the Department of Water and Power and the television station at Los Angeles by telling them over phone that he has dumped a gallon of AIDS-infected blood in one of the water reservoirs. He calls the County Board of Supervisors and tells them that if funds for testing sites are not released by them, one of the supervisors would be kidnapped, would be injected with the virus. He calls "the Federal Building, demanding release of a drug that people were smuggling in from China" (134). Lisa Garmire argues that "Dell's rage drives him to wish for more chaos, since revenge needs a target he can't clearly identify" (13). However, Dell's target is the apathetic administrative system prevalent in the 1980s in Southern California. Perhaps through his threats, he wants the system to care about the AIDS crisis that had killed thousands of gays including Marcus. Dell's target is once again Mother Evangeline, a white American woman in her mid-forties, who denounces homosexuals and says, '"Jesus would never have cured a man with AIDS, despite his record on leprosy. 'After all, there's limits, [...]. These homosexuals eat each other's feces. Do you think people like that deserve a miracle?'"(3). Ever since Dell has heard these words on TV, he has decided to kill her. Once he makes a call, "'Yeah, is Mother Evangeline there? Well, tell her there's a bomb in her church'" (10). Later on, wearing ghoul's clothes, Dell enters Evangeline's church and watches her speak:

> "My friends, my children," said Mother Evangeline, [...]. As her eyes scanned the faces of her sheep, she caught sight of the ghoul, [...]. "All our enemies are on the run," she declared, [...]. "The heathen and the pornographer, the whore and the sodomite. They are the ones who bring hell to earth, and it's time we sent them back where they came from." [...] "Ours is the kingdom, don't ever forget it. And thank God for AIDS. Sometimes He is a God of wrath before He is a God of love. And we are His army. Remember that next Tuesday. [...]" (136)

This is the rabid rightist's way of looking at homosexuals and AIDS. Dell smears turkey blood in the church office and then goes into hiding for fear of being arrested for such acts of vandalism. He stays in Steven's house where he sees that Heather, an employee at Shaw travel takes upon herself the responsibility of grooming his sister

Linda as her future colleague in the office. Dell feels that Linda is secure and he is free from family bondage. Thereafter his rage continues to grow. He gets caught up in the chaos again: "Did he know what he wanted? Not quite yet. He was still making this up as he went along, since the very first call to the water department. He astonished himself every step of the way. It was all he had anymore to prove he was still alive, the surge of unlikeness, the opposite of reason" (246). One morning armed with a gun hidden in his lap Dell leaves Steven's house uninformed, boards the bus to Mother Evangeline's. He keeps cool: "Anger wasn't part of it at all anymore. Anger might have veered him from the path. This was passionless, indifferent, not quite real" (269). In the church, he remains focused only to kill: "Dell pointed the gun at Mother, who threw out her hands to stop it, praying for once in her life. He shot directly into her face, no hate anymore, no reason" (272). After this, he gets confused as the congregation surges forward to catch hold of him: "Dell seemed perplexed, not having figured the next part out. It was really almost an afterthought that he put the gun in his mouth" (272).

Monette's portrayal of Dell as a murderer who eventually kills himself draws attention to the fact that clinging to the past inviolately and irreconcilably with obsessive grief and anger might arouse killer's instinct (both homicidal and suicidal) causing effacement of identity in HIV- positive people. This is at one level. At another level, Dell represents a drastic affirmation of identity in his crusade against a dominant community that chronically infuses persecution complex into gays and HIV- positive people.

Contrary to Steven and Dell, the third major character Sonny Cevathas, a Greek body-builder is an escapist, always denying the past and the present linked with his HIV-positive status, and instead fantasizes about a future free from AIDS. Sonny is a waiter and lives more or less in the Mercedes car that he has arbitrarily taken possession of from the family of his lover Ellsworth who had already died from AIDS. He is also a prime-time body-builder (athlete and aerobics dancer) at the gymnasium called The Body Works and depends on New Age literature: "The Body Works was Sonny's living room, his office, and his yard" (61). At the gym, he is the source of attraction for everybody: "There were a dozen regular Adonises in the class, but Sonny had the edge of being mascot. [...] It was Sonny the class watched"(61). His body language has sex appeal: "[...] he capered like figure on a Greek vase, erotic and in-the-body and far beyond it too" (61). In addition to these, "Sonny's youth and beauty were a magic circle" (62). That's why everybody watches him, and he enjoys seducing them even as he differentiates the physical (matter) from the spiritual (mind) from the perspective of the New Age philosophy - a differentiation that his late lover Ellsworth, he feels, was not aware of:

> [...], he stroked his vivid limbs in full view of a dozen others who could see they were lesser gods than he. Yet Sonny always gave them the chance, [...] even as far as going to bed once. After all, it often required the full body to put them in touch with the not-body. This, he had come to see, was where Ellsworth had failed him, by keeping Sonny's body at the objectified level of pure desire. If only Ellsworth could have broken through metaphysically, he never would have gotten sick at all. In his own way Sonny had truly loved Ellsworth and tried not to judge him. He understood that different men had different karmas to enact. But the last of the grief he felt was indistinguishable from a sort of moral posture, that a man made a journey of his own devising. (63-64)

In fact, Sonny's faith in New Age can be seen as a strategy to overcome his grief over Ellsworth's death and to deny his HIV-positive status. This is suggested as Sonny feels at the gym, "the sickness did not penetrate the walls of the Body Works [...]" (64). For him, the gym is "a sanctuary [...] where AIDS did not intrude, where people really meant it when they said they were feeling great"(64). For this reason, Sonny declines to go through the AIDS test following the death of Ellsworth: "He knew he had made the right choice not to be tested for the virus. The real test was the vast aliveness he felt at the end of Prime Time, gathering up his workout clothes and stuffing them in his gym bag, feeling a throb in his groin from the smell of his own sweat"(64). At any rate, he must deny his HIV-positive status and the threat of AIDS for his psychological and physical (sexual) survival. He must try to erase from his memories his past associated with the horrifying and fatal impact of AIDS on Ellsworth on the one hand, and the significance of the disease on his present on the other. That is why when his roommate Dirk Ainley develops AIDS-related symptoms such as white patches along the inner side of the lower lip and flu, Sonny flees out of the situation with pounding heart: "Sonny practically lurched from the room, hurrying out of the apartment as if he was late. He trotted down to the garage and pulled the Mercedes out, [...]. There was such a wall up between him and Ellsworth's illness that he didn't let the memories flood back in, refused to see again the white patches that foamed over Ellsworth's tongue, or hear the amulet phrase they had repeated over and over: 'Just the flu'" (100). He cannot face his past and therefore must run away. Ironically, Sonny can use Ellsworth's Mercedes 380 and cashmere sweaters and yet refuses to be reminded of his agonizing death from AIDS through Dirk's plight. He leaves the apartment and moves to Steven's house to stay there.

Sonny's denial of his HIV-positive status surfaces again at the time of his sexual union with Sean Pfeiffer, an extremely wealthy man who is six years younger than

Sonny's own father and is seduced by his beauty at the gym the Body Works. Sonny makes fun of safe sex when he chews and breaks the bulbous tip of the condom used by him and sucks out his cum:

> [...]. "Now you came in me twice," he said, staring at Sean with a passion that appeared to have no limits.
>
> "Very fucking hot," admitted Sean, always glad to see a new trick. "But are you sure you should do that?"
>
> "You mean is it safe?" Sonny gave a languorous shrug, as if the question was beneath him. "The stomach juices kill all that. Besides, you're a total top man, aren't you?"(185)

When Sean asks him about a crimson spot near his triceps, Sonny lies, '"It's a birthmark, why? You paranoid or something?"'(187). He knows that red spot is really Kaposi's sarcoma:

> Of course it wasn't a birthmark. A month now and it hadn't gone away, and the lymph node under it swollen like a golf ball. The only way out, he'd known all along, was to find again the river and source of his ancient fate. [...].
>
> [...]. The only part of his body still here was the flesh with which he would capture and enchant the beast beside him. Otherwise he was a hundred generations, beyond decay and pestilence. From now on it was he who would call down plagues. And Death, he saw as he fell into a slumbering swoon, Death was only for slaves. (192)

One day Sean gives Sonny two thousand dollars and seriously wants the latter to get his red spot checked up by a doctor. Sonny however is hurt and feels "as if he'd raped himself. He'd never done it for money"

(203). After this incident, "He was so sick of men, he could hardly breathe. He had a wild flash of understanding how sex criminals sometimes pleaded to have it cut off" (203). This reflects that Sonny's denial of and resistance to the threat of AIDS has almost become a part of his unconscious mind. He enters the shower, "where the last thing he expected was to come out clean" (203-04).

Yes, Sonny wants to rinse away his AIDS-associated past and present by turning to a channeler named Salou, an advocate of New Age philosophy. Salou authorizes Sonny's continuous denial of past and present in favour of a certain AIDS-free future. He tells Sonny that he is not gay and can get rid of gay disease: "'That will pass, [...] Once you leave the path. Your soul is too old to die young'" (234). Inspired by Salou, Sonny desperately wants to change his mind and to purify his body. In this way, he just wants to elude what he is then and now in relation to HIV/AIDS and to have a fresh life free from gayness and the disease in future. He discards his material belongings that represent his homosexual identity: "Before he went to bed he cleaned his house. Tossed in a Hefty bag his porno tapes, his poppers, butt plug, leather straps. Even his jockstrap. All the evidence he could gather of his carnal ride across the world of the body. He regretted none of it, missed none of it, as he dumped it all in the trash can at the curb. Just an immeasurable sense of relief" (234).

For Sonny, to forsake materialistic living that so far stood for his homosexuality and his HIV-positive status will result in cleansing and ushering in a new unblemished life. In doing so, he thinks that his sorrow will be reduced and his Kaposi's sarcoma beaten. He reasons under the influence of New Age: "If he wasn't gay anymore, perhaps he could reinvent being a boy from the bottom up" (253). Finally, in accordance with Salou's admonition not to put down roots, he leaves Steven's house to keep moving and "to break loose from all destination" (253). The figure of Sonny remains open-ended in the novel and suggests that he is non-committal to place and person, and is always in the run for a secure future never to be affected by AIDS. The novel communicates the message that there is futility of HIV-positive life in the acceptance of Sonny's strategy of coping with AIDS. Sonny's denial of his gay identity in order to be clear of HIV/AIDS, known then as a gay disease, might be viewed as his internalized homophobia. However, because of and not in spite of AIDS Sonny wants to deny his sexual identity. Monette wants his readers to see this.

Besides the major characters such as Steven, Dell and Sonny, there is a minor character named Ray Lee who is gay and subsequently dies of AIDS. He is a Korean working with Steven's travel agency. For Steven he is not sexual: "He seemed somehow above all that, androgynous and rarefied. He had even been some kind of monk for a while, or at least he'd gone to monk school. Steven had always considered him rather lucky, to be so removed from mantalk and the purely carnal" (122-23). This unmasculine portrayal of Ray is disturbing, since as Lisa Garmire rightly notes, "Unfortunately, Ray's effeminacy links together with his Asian-American identity, such that the representation of him in the novel comes dangerously close to a racial stereotyping of the Asian-American male as effeminized and as exotically non-Western"(20). This is overemphasized when the white American Steven sees AIDS-infected Ray's naked body thrashing back and forth on the bed: "He didn't seem to be in any pain. It was all rage. Startling because the Korean's demeanor had always been so placid. [...] Steven couldn't help but see his dick, long and uncut, the foreskin tapering generously like an anteater's snout. Steven blushed [...] wondering if uncut was the general rule for Asians. Surely not. They were so fastidious. *Shut up,* he screamed in his head" (238). However, in the figure of Ray, Monette suggests the unavoidability of body loss, desirelessness and non-identity leading to death that all HIV-positive people, including the three AIDS-infected widowers and their friends will have to face. Ray has been presented as the personification of AIDS. He invokes the AIDS stereotype. Ray symbolizes AIDS or what Yingling would have called, "the impossibility of speaking the condition of loss being written into (and onto) the body [...]: the whole problem of a disappearing body, of a body quite literally shitting itself away" (16).

Margaret, a copilot at Shaw travel, looks after the bedridden Ray in a motherly manner even as her colleague Heather initially gets scared, quits the job and later regrets for her behaviour. Though she is heterosexual, she helps all gay HIV-positive men, which is why her own love-life with Richard is disrupted. As Margaret puts it before Steven, "'*Richard*? [...] he thought he was going to get AIDS from the *turkey*. Richard and I are deader than Ray'" (254). Monette shows the usual phobic response to homosexual AIDS. Margaret unhesitatingly takes good care of Ray till his death. She represents matriarchy in a male homosexual and HIV-positive society. In her figure, Monette counters the notion of patriarchy in a heterosexual 'family' system.

Monette also deals with the role of a 'support group' known as "Gay and Lesbian Central" that meets every Thursday night in Los Angeles. Steven and Mark attend those meetings. Varieties of HIV-positive people gather there: "In fact they were all bizarrely different from each other, random as a planeload of refugees" (72). In this group, the problems faced by the infected are discussed and taken care of. Monette's intention here is to play down "family" that AIDS-infected people can do without in maintaining their identities. Thus, *Afterlife* projects the multidimensional aspects of the identities of the HIV-positive people in a counter-hegemonic mode.

Vance Bourjaily's *Old Soldier* (1990) deals with the death of a middle-aged gay man who has AIDS. It is written from the perspective of his older brother who, despite being straight, counters the homo-and-AIDS phobia that consequently sparks off a furious gun-battle in which his younger brother is shot at and severely injured. Joe McKay, a sixty-year-old soldier fights bravely to save the life of his fifty-five-year-old brother Tommy, a bagpiper in a New York country music bar who is gay and has just tested positive for AIDS. Apparently, the novel deals with the subject of encounter with the phobic notion of HIV/AIDS. Of course, it is more about AIDS phobia than about homophobia, which is only implied and not prominently displayed. The encounter however takes place not in the socially structured institutions or organizations, but in the woods, in the midst of nature. In so doing, Bourjaily suggests that phobias and sexual categories are present everywhere including the city and the country and are deeply rooted in the human psyche that needs to be drastically changed by individual's own rational participation in the act of resistance.

Bourjaily has chosen a campsite on a river in the Maine woods as the location to demonstrate his strategy of resisting stigma and homo-and-AIDS phobia. With the intention to fish, Joe goes to the site where he is received by his old friend Arnie who is "gatekeeper and campground manager" (92). The other campers at the site are twenty-six-year-old Carl Shumaker, his father John, his maternal uncle Doc Miles and two Pennsylvania country boys named Brad and Grady. All of them are listening to the radio commentary of a basketball match between the Boston Celtics and the Milwaukee Bucks. Subsequently, Tommy arrives there and joins them in a cheerless mood: "He seemed tired. [...]. There was some kind of pallor [...]" (126). This situation can be viewed in the following light: Joe, Arnie and the other campers enjoying sports represent a 'healthy' masculine world that is subsequently disturbed by the 'diseased' male presence symbolized by Tommy. Bourjaily also presents the dichotomy between the healthy and the diseased in terms of sexuality. Joe, Arnie and the campers are heterosexuals, and Tommy is homosexual. Bourjaily builds up this hegemonic notion and subsequently challenges it. However, his challenge takes place within the straight community itself as the story progresses. When others are gone leaving the two brothers to themselves, Tommy divulges to Joe that because of suffocation he fails to play as a participant in the bagpipe contest, '"I'd have run out of breath"' (128). He then reveals that he has tested HIV positive in a tone that is political, caustically humorous, is loaded with activist spirit at the same time:

> "[...] I've got it, Joe, the fairy-killer. God who loves us found a way to slap the wrists of bad little fairy boys, only the way he slaps, it breaks off your hand and the rest of you goes pouring out the stump. What's the dirty new four-letter word?"
>
> [..]
>
> "There can be a cure [...]. There's an army of people working on it."
>
> "Couple of squads. Joe, I know how you feel about the President. No matter what sorry specimen's in there, he's your commander-in-chief. I just wish Wrinkle Dick and Nancy didn't take the same attitude as God who loves us. [...]." (128-30)

Tommy is condemning the right-wing religious leaders, President Ronald Reagan and his wife Nancy whose heterosexual, pro-family and anti-gay attitude inflamed homophobia and aggravated deaths of thousands of gays from AIDS known then as a 'gay disease' in the 1980s in America. Tommy's present remark is just an extended version of what might be called his earlier sarcastic definition of AIDS –'"Dear old God's final solution to the sodomy problem"' (50). He regrets not to have been able to play the pibroch "Lament for the Children" in the contest. Through his music, he originally intended to memorialize his dead HIV-positive gay friends Bruno, Fletcher and Gary and to arouse a deep concern for the infected in the masses: '"I wanted the audience to mourn them with me, even if they didn't know they were doing it'" (130). His unfulfilled noble intention of waging a moral crusade for the gay cause points to his resistance to the dominant cultural feeling surrounding AIDS.

In 1990 when the novel was published, there was evidence of heterosexual AIDS. However, the popular perception in America was that AIDS was a gay disease. Bourjaily reveals this in the figure of Joe. Joe's wife Deedee who even crushes the photo of Tommy, since '"The big fat faggot's got a hole in his head"' (7), insists on divorce following her regular liaisons with Victor. Tommy suggests to Joe to have himself tested for AIDS:

> "Me?"
>
> "You've been sleeping with Deedee. She's been partying with Victor. How do you know who else big Vic parties with?"
>
> Joe seemed about to say something, changed his mind and kept it simple.
>
> "Life in the minefields."
>
> [..]
>
> Joe was turning out to be Mr. Hesitation himself. (49-50)

Ironically, Joe avoids the subject of heterosexual transmission of AIDS as though it is a total impossibility. His silence justifies the perception that only gay men get AIDS.

Tommy in his youth had married a woman named Holly. After a brief period of their marriage, he divorced her without knowing then that she was two months pregnant. Immediately after this, Joe has an affair with Holly. Later on, Holly gives birth to a son who is brought up by Joe. Joe calls the baby Little Joe who is now sixteen years old. In fact, Little Joe is the son of Tommy. That is why Tommy is '"the family man, Dean of Gays'" (55). Heterosexual Joe has married twice without any children. He is '"the childless macho man'" (55). However, "Joe had always loved Little Joe like his own. Matter of fact, the lad looked more and more like his uncle as he got older" (53). This is despite Joe's assertion that "'Little Joe's your kid all the way, Tommy, and I envy you. I surely do'" (53). Of course, by delivering Little Joe to Joe, the novelist is arguing for heterosexual foster parents as against gay parenting that did not find favour with the then US administration following AIDS in the 1980s.

Initially, Joe was not happy about Tommy being gay:

> By the time Tommy was fishing age, Joe was already in the army. Maybe Tom would have turned out different if he'd had a big brother at home. One of Joe's most troubling memories, [...], was of being nineteen, home on leave from the big war, [...]. Standing in the crowd, Joe heard a man say, "I hear that pretty blond one sucks a sweet dick."
>
> Joe had whirled, looking for the guy to hit, thought he saw who it was, but couldn't get to him. Joe had to get older before he learned to live with Tommy's being gay. Joe had had to serve with homosexual guys in the wars, and learn that some of them could soldier, to get his head straight about the matter. (10)

This indicates Joe's transformation from his notion of gayness as an 'acquired' condition to his understanding of homosexuality as a 'natural' thing. It is not his brotherly feeling that brings about this attitude change in him. His ability to appreciate the larger social practice of homosexuality brings in change in his notion. The campground conversation concerning Tommy's infection with AIDS arouses kindness in Joe who affectionately suggests, "'[...] think about moving in with me in Connecticut when we leave. I've got a lot of room now Deedee's ass is out of the way. You don't need to work, Tom. I'm making good money, and I get damn lonesome. It would do me good to have you around'"(130-31). Their talk is overheard by Carl Shumaker. Immediately after that, the entire scene is gripped by AIDS phobia. Through Tommy, Bourjaily starts his AIDS awareness campaign. Carl's father John will not listen to Tommy who says that '"you can't get AIDS from a toilet seat" (132) and that '"It only gets into your bloodstream where the skin is broken. Or with a needle"' (133). Despite Tommy's explanation, John remains unconvinced and still believes that AIDS is transmitted through shaking hands and through drinking from the same bottle. Astonishingly his brother-in-law Dr. Miles, a chiropractor, is terribly afraid: '"[...] I haven't read up on it. I do understand that it's a highly infectious disease, with one hundred percent fatalities"' (136). He does not like to read Tommy's pamphlet dealing with how AIDS is transmitted for fear of being infected through touching the booklet. This phobic situation is juxtaposed with counter-phobic state of affairs. Joe even without knowing the modes of HIV transmission hugs his brother, '"Come on, peckerbrain. If there was any reason not to, you'd have said so'" (134). Even Joe's friend Arnie is not afraid, and instead wants to ride the trailer along with the two brothers after knowing that Tommy has AIDS. He says to Joe about Tommy, "'Well, he can't give it to me, can he? Notice you're riding with him'" (141).

Tommy then has to read some lines aloud from a booklet written by an AIDS support group to Dr. Miles who finally says, "'Let me think about it'" (138). All these draw attention to the social perception of HIV/AIDS as stigma. The battle line is drawn. Readers watch a martial scene. In panic Brad and Grady burn Joe's camper, then leave the place immediately driving their vehicle as fast as possible. They are chased by Joe who angrily calls them '"Pennsylvania scumbags'" and '"cuntheads'" (140) suggesting their effeminacy. Bourjaily perhaps tries to indicate that those who cannot face AIDS are unmasculine. Arnie, in the meanwhile, stops Joe from pursuing them. He informs Joe that the police have already been called to deal with them on their way. In this incident, Joe is injured when shards of glass fall on his face. However, at this moment Doc Miles undergoes a change after reading the pamphlet. Simultaneously, John's attitude also changes as he says to Joe, "'Doc read that pamphlet Tommy left. He wants to tell Carl things are okay, not to worry. The boy's out of his head'" (142). Even Miles says, "'Is there anything we can do?'"(142). To all these, Joe's reply is "'You can fuck off'" (142).

However, stricken with panic Carl '"that thinks he's infected"' (137) lets out all the air from the tyres of Joe's truck and Tommy's motorcycle with the intention of keeping both brothers from communicating with each other quickly. In the meanwhile, Tommy is missing in the woods. While searching for his brother by canoeing through the rapids of the river, Joe hears rifle shots. Carl has shot Tommy to kill him, since he has AIDS. Joe pounces on Carl and gives him a blow that sends his rifle flying, starts kicking his ribs and finally puts him in the bear trap. Carl then says to Joe, "'It's your brother who's killing us all,' [...]. 'Don't you realize? He's the one you oughta lock up, Joe, he's got me infected. I know he does. Probably you, too'" (156-57). Later on Joe instructs John to contact the Ranger for unlocking the bear trap to get his son back.

Joe's concern is for Tommy who is bleeding profusely following a gunshot that has got through his ankle. AIDS cannot be a barrier in the fraternal bond as Joe feels *"he's my brother"* (155) and gets some blood on his hands while trying to stop the flow. Tommy advises him: '"Joe, your face. Where the glass got you. Don't wipe your face till your hands are clean"' (155).

Joe leaves Tommy alone for a while to make arrangement for transporting his wounded brother out of the woods. Tommy is in a reflective mood: "Now he started thinking about Joe. And Little Joe. The two people he loved in this world. Wondering about staying in Joe's house as he got sicker. Not liking that much. How messy he'd be. Hating the idea of telling Little Joe. Feeling a lot of fear. A lot of it, and not just for when the painkiller would wear off" (162). Tommy does not like to be a burden on his brother. Nor does he like the idea of being a mark of stigma for his own son who loves Joe more than Tommy. This however is not good enough reason for his mysterious disappearance from the novel. Perhaps Tommy dies by drowning himself in the river. This is suggested when Joe returns to the spot where Tommy was initially lying wounded and does not find any one:

> "Jesus," Joe said. [...]. "Tommy," he shouted. "Tommy."
>
> "He can't be gone," Doc Miles said.
>
> "He could have dragged himself," Joe said. There was a trail of disturbed leaves on the forest floor. They followed it to the river. There was blood on an exposed rock three feet out in the water.
>
> "Tommy," Joe yelled. "Tommy," and splashed out into the river, looking wildly downstream. There was nothing he could see downstream but water, and this time the tug of it against his legs was something fearful.
>
> "Oh, God," he said, turned, splashed back. "God, Tommy."
>
> Joe McKay slipped, fell to his knees on the riverbank, and wept. (164)

Kruger argues that Tommy's death signifies "a removal

of both AIDS and homosexuality" (160) and "the reaffirmation of an undisturbed, male, heterosexual space" (160). However, whether Tommy drowns himself or accidentally falls in the river remains a puzzle. Moreover, his death is a lingering, honourable one. Tommy is resurrected through Joe who observes his brother's death instantly and befittingly: "Then he waded into the river a few steps, set the bagpipe down in the water [...]" (166).

This memorialization of Tommy continues until the end of the novel. Little Joe is now called Joker, since "he was too big to be called Little" (167). Joker reminisces about his father as Joe asks him:

> "Missing your Dad?"
>
> "I never saw that much of him. Only in the last year or two - but I was starting to like him a lot. Sure I miss him. I wish he was here with us."
>
> "So do I." [...].
>
> [...]
>
> "He died a clean death, didn't he?
>
> "Yes."
>
> "His life wasn't all that clean, though."
>
> "Shut up, Joker. He had a lot of fun. He helped a lot of people. And people are going to be listening to his records for a while."
>
> [...]
>
> Joker felt like hugging him, so he did. (168-69)

Tommy's legacy will continue to be present in his non-existence. His perpetual spiritual presence in the novel will continue to change the attitudes of heterosexuals like John and Doc Miles who can give up their stigma-centric mindset towards persons living with AIDS. The removal of Tommy from the novel will work to reassure a certain space for gays and HIV-positive persons in heterosexual matrix. Tommy has become a consciousness that works to change the stereotypical human psyche. Of course, it is through Joe that he becomes all the more meaningful. It is Joe who confronts homo-and-AIDS phobia and makes everything happen.

The counter-hegemonic way of looking at HIV-positive identity is also seen in Christopher Davis's *Philadephia* (1993), which is based on the screenplay written by Ron Nyswaner. The film version of the book won an Oscar award. The novel is the story of a white American lawyer who faces discrimination for being gay and HIV positive and consequently, gets a lawsuit filed on his behalf by a Black American lawyer to see that justice is meted out to him. It critiques different forms of social discrimination such as homophobia, racism and class in general. In this larger context of differentiation, it looks at HIV-positive person in order to bring about positive changes in public attitudes towards the infected and the non-heterosexuals. It is written from a heterosexual perspective.

Andrew Beckett is "*the* star associate" (19) at the most prestigious Philadelphia law firm of Wyant, Wheeler. Ironically, "[...] he often said the best lawsuits were ones that didn't happen [...]" (45). His observation reflects that he loves peace. He has been living for eight years with his gay lover Miguel Alvarez who is from Spain, teaches at the Institute of the Arts. He has "full-blown AIDS" (13). He has been assigned a very important case by his firm. This is "the high point" of his young career (32). However, the lesion on his forehead becomes visible and is discovered by Mr. Kenton, one of the firm partners. Immediately after this, the files of his final draft of the Highline complaint on his computer, files that are meant to be served on time, disappear. Andrew is dismissed by Charles Wheeler, the main partner on grounds of what the latter calls, '"A kind of stupor, a fogginess, a lack of focus'" (73). Andrew however knows that the file was deliberately misplaced to discover a clue to fire him. The real reason for his termination is his infection with AIDS.

Andrew wants to sue Wyant, Wheeler for discrimination and to fight for his dignity, for his job and for justice. He meets many attorneys to represent him, "And almost always the attorney washed his or her hands thoroughly as soon as Andrew left" (83). Despite their behavioural pattern born out of stigma attached to the disease, he refuses to give up. Finally, he meets Joe Miller who is a personal injury lawyer in a small firm, and who gets his clients through television advertisements. He reasons, "He's black, so he understands discrimination, and he's not a bad lawyer, [...]" (84). The novelist is tagging the stigmatization of HIV-positive people on homo-and-AIDS phobic grounds on to the racial discrimination of Black Americans and thereby targets the social structures of discrimination. Earlier in the novel, Joe has been shown to have experienced this racism: "[...] he was black and there were very few black partners at major law firms, a situation that Joe did not think was going to change in the near future"(8). Racism is stressed once again in the book when Anthea Burton, a black paralegal at Wyant, Wheeler appears as witness in Andrew's trial. She confesses that she feels '"discriminated against'" in the firm (163). As reported to her by Lydia, Mr. Wheeler's secretary, Charles does not like her "large, long, dangling earrings" (163). In response to Joe's question, Burton says, '"Apparently, Mr. Wheeler felt that they were too 'ethnic.'[...] Mr. Wheeler would like me to wear something smaller, less garish, 'more American.'"'(163). She then adds, '"[...] my earrings *are* American - African-American."'(164). Hence, the thrust of the novel is discrimination in its institutionalized form.

Initially Joe, whose heterosexuality and patriarchy have been emphasized, refuses to represent Andrew on homo-and-AIDS phobic grounds. This is revealed as he calls on his doctor with apprehension, "'[...] there was this man with AIDS in my office and I shook his hand and with the new baby and everything...'" (94). The physician gives him a lesson on how AIDS is transmitted. As is usual with all HIV/AIDS narratives, the novel at this point tries to raise AIDS awareness. At home, his wife Lisa tries to dispel his homophobic attitude by referring to her familiarity with gay people who are her relatives, such as her cousin, aunt and so on. Joe instantly asks her to stay away from them. Despite his anti-gay mindset, Joe subsequently becomes Andrew's lawyer when he understands that discrimination is unjust: "God, I hate this case, [...] but the guy is right" (106). The "guy" refers to Andrew who says to Joe in the law library, "'[...] AIDS is protected as a handicap under law not only because of the physical limitations it imposes, but also because the prejudice surrounding AIDS exacts a social death which precedes the actual physical one'" (105-06). This takes place at a moment when he learns that Andrew being turned down by all lawyers decides to represent himself in his case. Subsequently, Joe gets summons issued for Charles Wheeler as he "did believe in the law [...]; he could say truthfully that he took Andrew's case for the principle, not the money" (111).

From this time onwards, the novel's focus shifts from Andrew to Joe. As the story progresses, Joe emerges as the central character of the novel even if the action revolves round Andrew who seems to be the main character. The story's action is furthered because of Joe. Andrew is relegated to a marginal position, is almost reduced to the position of a spectator. He is shown as someone having the will to live and fight despite being HIV positive, as someone struggling for his survival with dignity. For example, to "forget the nasty little virus"(16) inside him and "the lesions" on his body while receiving treatment from Dr. Gillman in her clinic, he always listens to classical music by turning on his Walkman. In order to make himself psychologically strong he engages in tasks that fill him with positive energy and with the spirit of adventure. He reads once more James Joyce's *Ulysses* to get lost in its "meandering complexities" (114). To make himself feel lighter he does meditation, closes his eyes and repeats continuously the woman's voice on the tape: '"I can heal myself"' (115). Even though his health is seriously deteriorating day by day, he reads law books to find out strong points in his favour in the ongoing case. His unyielding fighter's spirit is reflected in his conversation with his lover Miguel:

> "I'm not ready," Andrew repeated.
>
> "Say it!" Miguel suddenly yelled.
>
> "To die," Andrew said very quietly.
>
> "Do you think I'm ready for it?" Miguel shouted. "I hate this shit!"
>
> [...]
>
> "I'm just scared," Andrew said. "I am so terribly scared."(190)

Caught up in the struggle between the will to live and the fear of death, Andrew organizes an opera show at home, dances in the gay party with Miguel to the tunes of the music "it's Madison time" and gets "totally immersed in the moment"(200). Towards the last part of the novel, he knows, '"There's a possibility I won't be around for the end of this trial" (206). He therefore speaks to Joe about his will for some charities and for Miguel. He requests Joe to help his lover after his death.

With the help of Miguel, Andrew receives the IV treatments at home through implanted catheter. Even then he wants to celebrate his desire for life and love as he listens to the French music by Giordano: "Inside Andrew danced, he danced for life, he danced for music, he danced for love, he danced for hope, and as the music expanded and grew he danced more freely, unhooking his IV, and he danced for death. He was not ready, but he was getting there, it was becoming a reality, a visible part of his life, and he started the aria again, singing along in parts; 'Live! ... I am life! ... I am love!'" (208-09).

He wants justice even though heterosexuals see his lawsuit as a gay rights issue. This is evident when Andrew meets an angry mob outside the court after the first day of his trial. Andrew speaks into the microphone to answer questions from TV reporters. To the question "'Do you see this as a gay rights issue?'", Andrew's answer is "'I'm not political, [...]. I just want what's fair, what's right'" (154). To the query "'But you are gay, aren't you?'", his retort is "'I don't see how that's any of your business, [...] but yes, I am'" (154). Andrew can assert his gay identity audaciously, disregarding the reaction of the angry mob. As a witness, he is uncompromisingly truthful in the court as he confesses that he is gay. He also explains, '"You don't bring your personal life into a law firm"' (213). His straightforward admission of fact even makes the defense lawyer Belinda Conine realize that the charges of incompetence and sabotage on Andrew are false: "'I hate this case,' Ms. Conine whispered [...], 'and I hate it when clients lie to me.' Ms. Conine was beginning to think that Joe and Andrew were right" (224). Despite having developed constant vomiting, terrible weakness and eyesight and concentration problems, Andrew adamantly wants the trial to continue: "He would not give up until he saw Charles Wheeler on the stand" (228). He watches Charles appear as witness and lie under oath to the court. Charles does not confess that Andrew was fired because of his HIV-positive status and gayness. He rather says that Andrew was dismissed because he wanted to benefit from the system without following the system's rules. Andrew collapses in the course of the trial, is subsequently hospitalized till his death and is not seen in the court till the last proceedings and verdict that go in his favour. Joe alone is seen in the court as though it is his victory. For Andrew, "his fight was over, his time was over, all there was left to do was leave" as he says, '"Miguel, I'm ready"' (245). Then he dies. Andrew's is a righteous fight both at individual and social levels for living and dying with dignity, despite being HIV positive.

This shows that Andrew's role is emotionally charged, whereas Joe is in the forefront of action. Initially, Wyant, Wheeler tries to defend itself by adopting the strategy of first overwhelming and then intimidating Joe. It assigns five lawyers to the case, and the chief litigant is Belinda Conine. It even influences Judge Garnett to be on its side. Garnett being heterosexual was also in its favour. However, Joe's threat to expose the corrupt practices of the legal establishment in the press compels Judge Garnett to be judicious. Considering the worsening health condition of Andrew, Joe expedites the process of interviewing witnesses and of obtaining copies of relevant documents, whereas the defense litigators' tactic is to delay the trial inordinately so that the plaintiff will not survive to see his case. Through press conferences Joe pressurizes the defense counsellors to get ready for immediate trial. Within one day, the selection of jury is made, and the trial begins next day. In fact, Joe effectively proves his prowess as a lawyer by raising baffling questions to his witnesses, even though his pleading strategy counts on Andrew's briefs on various legal points coupled with the witnesses' testimony. Through his tactical skill he could make law firm partner Kenton expose himself before the jury that the latter hates homosexuals, is already aware of the difference between a lesion and a bruise. Using his superb legal acumen, he establishes that Andrew has not infected Miguel with AIDS and that the latter is an excellent lawyer, is unquestionably trustworthy, is impeccably honest. Joe refutes all charges made by defense lawyers on Andrew. He proves that Charles is homophobic, believes in discrimination, be it based on sexuality, race, class, or HIV/AIDS.

The most important thing about Joe is that he is the only character who undergoes the attitudinal transformation that is so crucial to the action of the novel. Joe has been portrayed as hardcore heterosexual, gay-hater and homophobe. He represents patriarchy. Through his character, the novel is able to establish successfully a location with which the readers can identify. His anti-gay mindset has already been revealed when AIDS-infected Andrew meets him to represent the latter in the lawsuit. It is emphasized once again when Joe shouts at law student Mark who being a gay wants to date with him as the latter thinks him to be a homosexual, while seeing him on television in connection with Andrew's trial: "'I ought to kick your faggoty little ass for you!'"(170). Grabbing Mark's jacket he then says, "'Don't you know this is exactly the kind of bullshit that makes people hate you guys?'"(171). Later on Joe checks with his wife if he is looking like a gay, "'Is there some kind of expression I've picked up from Beckett? Some kind of attitude I've unconsciously adopted? Am I walking different?'" (172). His feeling can be juxtaposed with that of Charles Wheeler who expresses his disgust for homosexuals through jokes. For example, his question '"How does a faggot fake an orgasm?"' is followed by the answer '"He spits on your back'"(214). The novel shows that though Joe is black, belongs to the middle class, he shares his anti-gay sensibility with his defendant Charles Wheeler who is white, comes from the upper class because both of them are heterosexuals, despite their racial and class divisions. In fact, heterosexuality is the site of resistance to homosexuality. In the early 1990s when the book was written, heterosexual-AIDS was there in America. However, it was overlooked because of homophobia that continued to preoccupy the people. Despite the demand for anti-discriminatory behaviour towards overt homosexuals, the HIV/AIDS epidemic that killed mostly gays in the 1980s in America was seen as a justification for homophobia. This historical situation is evident in the book. The public response to the first day of Andrew's trial outside the court was one of war between homosexuality and heterosexuality:

> [...] Gay activists shouted, "Hey! Hey! Ho! Ho! Homophobia's got to go!" They were countered by "No rights for sodomites," and, from a small group [...]: "Death to faggots." When a preacher saw Andrew he shouted, "God created Adam and Eve, not Adam and Steve!" Even worse were some of the signs being carried: "God will not *allow* science to cure AIDS" and "GAY = Got AIDS Yet?" were just two of them. (154)

The novel therefore announces overt homosexuality in a heterosexual society. This is suggested in the final victory of Joe who undergoes transformation in his attitude to HIV-positive people and gays.

Joe's attitude change is the effect of his deeper understanding of racial, class and sexual discriminations in the course of the trial. This is shown as he responds to the question of the television reporter, Angela who, immediately after the first day of the trial, wants to know if homosexuals deserve special treatment: "'Angela, we're standing in Philadelphia, the City of Brotherly Love, the birthplace of freedom, where our Founding Fathers authored the Declaration of Independence. I don't remember that glorious document saying all *straight* men are created equal. I could have sworn it says, 'All men are created equal''"(155). In fact, herein lies the justification of the title of the novel. The situation also reminds Joe of the black rights movement: "How many years earlier would these same people, or people like them, have reacted the same way to the thought of equal rights for blacks?"(157). The civil rights movement of the Black

Americans in the late 1950s is juxtaposed with the gay rights movement in the late 1960s and 1970s.

Joe's transformation can also be seen as he launches a new TV commercial that reads: '"Are you tired of having doors shut in your face, just because you're disabled? You know you can do the job but they won't give you a chance? There's nothing you can do, right? Wrong! You don't have to settle for closed doors and a cloudy future just because you're physically, emotionally, or mentally challenged, or because of your sex, race or sexual orientation"' (191). He participates and even dances in a gay party organized by Andrew. After the party is over, Joe closely watches his client Andrew attach himself to an IV and, for a moment, is lost in a rational, just reflection: "for the very first time since he had known him he did not think 'gay man,' he just thought 'man who is dying.' And if he had been able to articulate it, he would have thought 'friend'" (206).

The most significant change in Joe is seen when Andrew ignores his instructions concerning questions to be raised and answers to be given in the next proceeding of the court. He instead turns up the volume of his stereo asking Joe to join him in listening to Madeleina. After sometime as he wants to look at the questions and answers, Joe is not interested in them anymore: "He could not think about them himself; all he could think of was how brave Andrew was and how much knowing Andrew had changed his own life" (208). After Joe wins the case, he goes to the hospital to celebrate their victory. However, he watches a dying Andrew: "He could not believe how much he cared for this man, the man who had taught him more about prejudice than he had learned before in his lifetime, the man who had taught him so much about the law, the man who had taught him so much about life" (243). Finally, as he holds Andrew's hand, "he remembered the time he was upset even shaking Andrew's hand. You son of a bitch, he thought, you have really made me care about you" (243).

In addition to Andrew's story, the counter-hegemonic note is seen in the story of Andrew's AIDS doctor Gillman. Dr. Gillman with the help of her defence lawyer who subsequently died of AIDS has "fought hard and won" against a lawsuit filed by her neighbours and landlord who "wanted her out because her patients were posing a 'mortal threat' to the community" (11).

The counter-dominant stand in the novel is also seen in the depiction of Melissa Benedict, a paralegal who contracted HIV during a blood transfusion immediately after giving birth to her second child. Benedict subsequently develops Kaposi's Sarcoma (KS). She says to the court that Kenton knew how KS looked like: "'Every time he came into contact with me, he'd get this look on his face. I called it the 'Oh God' look, as in 'Oh God, here comes that woman with AIDS'" (161). This revelation proves that Kenton first recognized KS on Andrew's forehead and that Kenton was the main conspirator to have him fired. When Benedict is cross-examined by the defense counselor, she says, "'I do not consider myself any different from everyone else who has this disease: I'm not guilty, I'm not innocent, I'm just trying to survive'" (162). Here the novel attempts to collapse the opposition between the "guilty" and the "innocent victim" in hegemonic HIV/AIDS discourse and thereby tries to establish that HIV/AIDS can happen to anyone.

In its portrayal of the responses of Andrew's family, the novel also counters the stereotypical notion of the dominant community. Knowing fully well that his private life (specially his gayness) would be highlighted in the proceedings of the court, Andrew seeks the approval of his family members. Andrew's mother Sarah says, '"Go ahead, fight for your rights"' (138). His father Bud says, "'[...] Andy, the way you've faced this whole thing, you and Miguel, with so much courage, your mother and I have been so impressed'"(139-40). Even his brother Matt, who had taken years to accept Andrew's gayness, says, "'Hey, you're my brother,' [...]. 'That's all that matters! What are those bastards going to say about you? That you're gay? Hell, I knew that before you did'" (140). All of them are ready to be witnesses. Of course, in almost all HIV/AIDS narratives, the family always supports HIV-positive people regardless of their sexual orientation. Facing the people's hostile response to homosexuality outside the court at the end of the first day of the trial, Andrew's mother Sarah says to a TV reporter, "'This is a world filled with wars, famine, poverty, homelessness. And people make a fuss because two men, or two women, want to live together, or make love. It all seems kind of silly, doesn't it?'"(157).

In the character of Lisa, Joe's wife the novel seeks to demonstrate its attempt to attack the stereotypical notion of human sexuality:

> [...]. "What is it you find so disgusting about two men making love?" She started unbuttoning Joe's pajama top.
>
> God, Joe thought [...]. "A guy putting his dick in another guy's mouth. It's just disgusting."
>
> Lisa kissed Joe's chest, nuzzling a little. "Okay, so help me with this one. Is it disgusting to put your penis into someone's mouth? Or is it disgusting to take someone's penis in your mouth?" She worked her way down to his stomach, then said, "I'm just curious," then went a little lower.
>
> This definitely had possibilities, Joe thought. "Which answer will get me what I want?" he said.
>
> Lisa stopped short, pulled herself up and put her head on pillow.
>
> "Was that the wrong answer?" Joe asked.
>
> "Yeup. Good night."(173-74)

This is a crucial scene in the novel. Lisa is heterosexual. Even then, she loves the homosexual. Lisa is an artist. So is Miguel. This is clear when Joe just before the above scene says to his wife, '"You know, Beckett's 'lover,' as he calls him, is an artist too"' (173). They differ only in their gender. Lisa is called wife, can procreate and therefore is socially acceptable and desirable. Miguel is called 'lover,' cannot reproduce and hence is socially unacceptable and undesirable. Both of them however are erotically the same. Their sexual desire and pleasure are the same. Therefore, discrimination on grounds of sexual orientation must be abolished. This is the message of the scene. Even as this scene helps Joe minimize much of his homophobia, it also works to bring about transformation in the readers. In fact, the novel ends not with pity but with a deeper understanding that works to dissolve discrimination.

Charlotte Watson Sherman's *Touch* (1995) is about how a thirty-five-year-old black HIV-positive straight woman copes with the trauma caused by the disease. The novel is written from the perspective of a heterosexual Black American woman. Unlike the above three novels, it deals primarily with heterosexual AIDS, even though there are very few instances of homosexual AIDS in the book. Of course, by 1995 when the novel was written, heterosexual AIDS was an established phenomenon in America. The novel focuses on the ways and practices of overcoming fear of the disease by the diseased themselves. Its counter-hegemonic strategy not only includes resistance to AIDS phobia but also involves the demand for the HIV-positive mother's right to give birth to her baby. The novel seeks to critique the cultural notion of the clinical as the most rational thing in health/disease discourse. The novel is the story of Rayna Sargent, a black woman who is diagnosed as HIV positive just at a time when she discovers that she is in love with a man named Theodore.

Rayna Sargent works as a telephone crisis-line counsellor at Central Hospital's Viewridge Mental Health Clinic, Seattle, Washington. She listens to "people's emotional problems over the telephone" (25). Initially, she has been portrayed as someone who has internalized 'fear.' She is afraid of having "someone get too close to her" (42) because her long five-year marriage with Carl Broussard ended in a divorce. She is equally afraid of giving birth to a child because she, being an adopted child or daughter of Circe and Car following the mental illness of her mother, feels that the child may be as "schizophrenic" (42) as her mother was. This reflects her highly sensitive and rational mind. Having chosen art as her life, Rayna has been living alone happily for some years. She shares her feelings, ideas and problems with C'Anne and Novel Lewis, her two friends who also work with her in the same place. C'Anne is a family person, and Novel is a divorcee.

In the first chapter of the novel, AIDS phobia is shown in the figures of both Novel and Rayna. Initially, for fear of being stigmatized Novel Lewis, a psychotherapist refuses to collaborate with Rayna in making art pieces for the show intended for an AIDS hospital called Bailey-Boushay House: "'AIDS? Who's going to see our work? I need to get my name out there. What if people think I've got AIDS? The only people going inside that place won't have art on their minds"' (6). For her, the House is meant for people who are going to die, and her participation could bring her '"bad luck"' (7). Even though Rayna persuades Novel to be part of the show, she herself is initially scared when she meets the HIV-positive gay artist Ricky Adonio in the Bailey-Boushay reception: "She had been afraid of Ricky. Afraid to touch him, afraid to be near him, breathing the air he breathed" (18). Immediately after this, Rayna feels guilty: "A snake's tail of shame coiled itself inside her belly. She could feel its poison sinking deep inside her bones, oozing into the core of her soul" (18). Sherman shows here the evolution of individual perception and awareness concerning AIDS.

In the second chapter, AIDS phobia is countered. The response of Novel and Rayna to Latosha Briggs shows this. In her clinic, Rayna as a black woman is asked to handle the case of Latosha Briggs, an HIV-positive black woman who, without her written consent, was forced to undergo abortion and sterilization by Dr. Van Home, whose argument was that the latter would give birth to an AIDS baby. Prior to this, Latosha was not given any counselling and was only shown the picture of the tormented life of an HIV-positive baby by psychiatrist Dr. Mencken. Subsequently, at another hospital, she learnt about the fifty-fifty possibility of giving birth to an HIV-negative baby on her part. However, she could not get pregnant again. Now she is in the last stage of AIDS, and her family ascribes her present condition to the stress of the abortion. Her sister develops depression following the stress of looking after everyone including her own children. Latosha has filed a suit against the hospital for discrimination, for causing mental suffering and for having abortion and sterilization performed without her consent. Rayna's immediate response to the case is somewhat conciliatory: '"Well, I have to go call the woman's sister now, try to calm her down and get her to get counseling somewhere else"'(32). However, Novel is very rebellious: '"I don't care if it's AIDS, Raid, or whatever. None of these doctors have the right to sterilize anybody who doesn't want to be sterilized. And if he did it, he's gonna pay for it"' (32). The novel moves back and forth between activism and fear of AIDS.

The Briggs case fans racist feeling. One day two black women from an activist group called the Prejudice Posse vandalize the hospital office by throwing on desks, papers, Rayna and the receptionist Jenny a vial of red liquid. They want others to believe that the red liquid is Latosha's AIDS-tainted blood. Even though Jenny gets hysterical and sobs for fear of being infected with AIDS, Rayna who has also the patches of red on her blouse and shoulder shouts, "'We can't do anything about Latosha Briggs. Why would you hurt us? Go after the doctors...'" (37). Somehow, she feels that the red liquid is not blood. She chases the vandals only to meet them face to face. Sherman here juxtaposes AIDS phobia that one succumbs to on the one hand and the audacity to face it on the other. Even as Rayna tries to convince them that she does not have any hand in the hospital's decision-making and therefore must not be targeted, they say, "'They would do the same thing to you if you ended up pregnant with AIDS. Would you be able to keep working for those fascists as if nothing was wrong then'" (41). To Rayna's question, "'Is this the only way you can find to make your point?'" (41), their answer is "'Yeah, you could say that, [...]. At least we know they are thinking about how they treat women with AIDS at your hospital, more than they ever have before. And that's the best point we can make'" (41). The black activist's stand is reminiscent of the spirit behind the protest made by the AIDS Coalition to Unleash Power (ACT UP) to end the AIDS crisis in the early years of the epidemic. Within a few days, this activist group holds protest rally in front of the clinic carrying placards: "[...] STOP RACIST STERILIZATIONS [...] HUG SOMEONE WITH AIDS [...] POSITIVE WOMEN FOR LIFE" (54). An older woman speaks to Rayna who is then on her way to take the elevator to reach her office room:

> "Daughter, we know you ain't no part of this mess," [...]. "But we could sure use your help. [...] some of us are carrying the HIV virus in our veins. [...]. Latosha is just about dead herself. We want to fight this thing with the clinic in her name and in the names of us all. [...]. People are afraid of us, not because of our protests or our marches [...] because we represent what could happen to them. They're afraid to work with us, to sit by us, [...]. They're even afraid to touch us. Afraid to touch us in a time when we need human touch most of all. You don't have to make love to us, just hold our hand. Tell us you know you don't

> understand how it feels, but you care how we feel. [...] You think you could do that for us, for your sisters?"(56-57)

The activist stand challenges the hegemonic perception of the disease as stigma. It tries to humanize AIDS. The options left for the diseased are either to die or to protest. The first option is cowardly, since it succumbs to the dominant ideology. The second one assures dignity of living. The 'human touch' for the HIV- positive people, which AIDS activists are struggling to have, is perhaps what the novel is about. In fact, the novel tries to make the disease palpable, to put a human face on the epidemic. Herein lies the justification of the title of the novel. Rayna gives her considered opinion to the older woman of the group: '"I'll think about it,' Rayna said, softly. 'But if you want help, you're going about it the wrong way. [...]. Throwing blood on people and telling them it's got AIDS is wrong"' (57). This reveals her unprejudiced mind. However, she does not like to dwell on this issue now. Rather, she is interested to begin a new relationship with Theodore Massey, an X-ray technician at the hospital, a relationship that C'Anne had deliberately been pressing Rayna to enter into to have freedom from her loneliness. Rayna speaks to Theodore, and gradually both of them come closer to each other within months.

Against the backdrop of AIDS activism, Sherman chooses to present Rayna's love affair. As the novel progresses, it will be noticed that the AIDS activism is the externalization of Rayna's mind that she fails to fathom right now. The novel thus has two plots interwoven into each other. Before their meeting, Rayna, who in the past had sex with a stranger on a train, with a minister in the church, with Matthew, with her high school maths teacher and with a sculptor, has decided to practise abstinence for fear of AIDS: "'With all of this talk about AIDS [...] I'm thinking about giving up sex myself. I have to turn myself into some kind of investigator every time I get with somebody new. It's such a hassle'" (62). Therefore, before having sex with Theodore, that too, after almost a two-year period of abstinence, she insists on using a condom:

> "I don't make love without a condom," Rayna had told him.
>
> [...]
>
> "Where's the romance in putting on a rubber?" he had asked.
>
> "We could make it a part of foreplay," she had responded. "But you know, I never think about romance when I'm scared about getting AIDS."
>
> "I take good care of myself and I know I don't have AIDS," he had said.
>
> "Have you been tested?"
>
> "I don't need no test to tell me what I already know. I don't got it."
>
> "But I know we've both had sex with other people, unless you're telling me that at thirty-eight years old, this would be your first time?" Rayna had asked unbelievingly.
>
> "I haven't been intimate with that many people, have you?" he had asked defensively.
>
> "It doesn't matter how many people we've been intimate with. When we sleep with each other, it's like we're sleeping with all of the people we've both gone to bed with. If we're together six months from now, we can both get tested, and if we're negative and monogamous and you aren't using IV drugs, then we can stop using the condoms. But until then, I can't enjoy sex when I'm worrying about a virus running wild in my body. So I won't have sex without using condoms."

> "Well, I can't feel anything with a rubber on. I don't want to use 'em." "Well, you can't feel anything when you're dead either," Rayna had told him [...]. (67-68)

Sherman attempts to disseminate safe sex message preferably among Black or African American men who see condom use, as Patricia Hill Collins observes, "as interfering with their pleasure and challenging a view of Black masculinity that glorifies sexual virility" (292). Often heterosexual black men's masculine identity is understood as something that exercises control over black women's femininity. Sherman tries to subvert this notion particularly in the context of HIV/AIDS, and thereby celebrates identity of "strong" African American women who can defy being sexually, economically exploited and used by heterosexual black men. She is in fact making a case for women's empowerment in their sexual relationships with men, given the threat that HIV/AIDS poses. Sherman does this deliberately even as in the novel through her character she pronounces, "'Black women are womanists, not feminists'" (36). The novelist also draws her readers' attention to the fact that in the epidemic situation of HIV/AIDS, autonomy of sexuality can be constructed and maintained. In this context, Collins's argument may be relevant:

> Individual choice lies at the heart of any long-range solutions to HIV/AIDS. On the one hand, individual African American women and men can construct their own sexuality and that of their partners as sites of control and domination. When heterosexual men, for example, demand sexual intercourse without a condom, they become part of the HIV problem, whether or not they are infected with the HIV virus. When heterosexual women trade sexual favours for material gain without practicing safe sex, they too are part of the problem. On the other hand, when individual

> African American women and men strive to develop honest bodies and to reclaim the erotic as a site of freedom, and love as a source of affirmation for self and others, they challenge the spread of HIV/AIDS. (290)

This is reflected in the sexual love between Rayna and Theodore, "Rayna took the thin layer of latex Theodore held in his hand like a gift and gently rolled it over his penis with her tongue. Then on and off through the night as they each opened the closed doors inside of themselves and revealed that naked place outside the body where the act of making love, the sex of the sex, would take them, only then did Rayna catch a glimpse of the color of Theodore's soul [...]" (71).

Latex use and HIV-positive pregnancy are very much emphasized in the novel. Obviously, Sheman's target audience is heterosexual Black Americans. There was a sharp rise in HIV infection among Black American women in the 1990s when the novel was written. Most of the women were very poor, infected with AIDS through heterosexual contact and diagnosed as HIV positive only after their pregnancies. At a very young age, some women had sex mostly with older men and found it difficult to persuade their partners to use condoms. Some earned money in this way to support their dependents such as old parents and minor children. Collins writes, "They knew about HIV/AIDS but felt virtually powerless to take the steps needed to protect themselves from infection. Because they had so little control over other aspects of their lives, they felt that if God wanted them to get AIDS, then they resigned themselves to getting it" (291).

One day Theodore tells Rayna about a lump on her neck. Her regular gynaecology doctor refers her case to Dr. Slope, an infectious disease specialist who wants to do ELISA test and Western blot test to see if Rayna has been infected with AIDS. Rayna by now is sick of listening to anyone talking to her about AIDS, ever since she has experienced the Briggs case and the Prejudice Posse. In line with the convention of all HIV/AIDS narratives, this novel also offers AIDS awareness messages through Dr. Slope. Rayna is overconfident that she would never have AIDS, "She had been practicing safe sex for several years and had only slipped a few times. There was no way in the world she could have AIDS. How could this be happening to her?"(80). When she is told that she is HIV positive, she slumps in the chair. This is followed by her silent recitation of her litany of gripping fears: "*The fear of air, the fear of bacteria, the fear of beards and beds, the fear of being afraid, the fear of being alone, the fear of being bound, the fear of being beaten, the fear of being buried alive*" (83). She is seized by "*the fear of everything*" (85).

This fear is accelerated by her second HIV test that also proves positive. She becomes very moody and withdraws into herself in her office. She avoids Theodore for weeks without telling him about her HIV- positive status. She does not even speak to Novel and C'Anne. She does not respond to any phone call for weeks together. Her life is devoid of meaning all on a sudden, "as if she were living in a dream. Each step, each breath, each sweep of her arms through the air felt accentuated and unreal" (91).

Rayna tries to know more about the disease by using the AIDS hotline. The photos of AIDS patients do not give her "the courage and strength to fight the disease she had thought they would" (96). A deep sense of self-annihilation overwhelms her:

> [...] the thought of lying in a hospital bed concentration-camp thin with those awful spots all over her body made her weep.
>
> No, she would kill herself first. She would have to do it before she got too sick. (97)

She blames herself for her past sex life: "Every face and member of the men she had bedded, every musky scent, every wisp of body hair. The moans, the shouts of joy, the ache once they had gone. [...] All of those sensations and smells came back to Rayna with the force of an accusatory finger pointing in her face" (99). However, she feels, '"No. I don't deserve this. I'm not guilty. I'm not"' (99). She now realizes the plight of the HIV-positive painter Ricky who is now living in Bailey-Boushay, an AIDS hospital for which both of them had once contributed the slides of their arts. Sherman dissolves the differences between homosexually and heterosexually transmitted AIDS, perhaps to suggest the non-gendered and non-discriminatory significance of the disease. Rayna goes to the hospital to meet Ricky. She first discloses her HIV-positive status to him, as "We sat and held hands like lovers" (100). Ricky also tells her about his experience of the disease, '"this virus [...] takes away everything that you love'" (100). Rayna feels she can no longer keep her disease to herself, "She felt that the weight of her secret might kill her otherwise. [...] She was growing weary of the lies she was telling, tired of feeling as if she were some kind of criminal because she had a disease"(109). Her home feels "like a grave" as she cannot "let anyone come over" and as she does not "dare go anywhere" (109). In the process, she begins to believe she is "going insane" (110). She deliberately keeps awake at night, since "Sleeping now reminded her of death. The thought of closing her eyes terrified her" (110). Finally, she tells Novel about her infection with AIDS. Rayna then experiences her mental evolution from fear to boldness as Novel with love holds the former protectively inside her arms, weeps and affectionately listens to the story of her agony. She says, '"You know, when I first got my test results back and they were positive, I just wanted to die. I didn't care anything about living with this disease. I just wanted to die. But now, I just want to live"' (116). She wants to have hope and happiness as she records her feeling in her journal:

I wish I could stand in the center of the world

> surrounded by a gospel choir in golden robes, [...] lifting me up in the arms of their belief, their voices rising like saviors to the heavens. I wish I could turn this sorrow into a blessing. I wish when I looked inside the hollow of my spirit, a startling of hope would rise inside me fluttering for the first time up through the bitterness of my soul breaking it down into something sweet like hope like forgiveness like salvation.
>
> I wish I could feel anything other than the emptiness I feel when I think about my spirit and ask god, why me? (117-18)

As suggested by Novel, Rayna then plucks up the courage to attend the Positive Women support group's meeting where she shares her feeling of being HIV positive with others:

> "[...] I don't know how I got this thing and I don't know who I got it from [...]. I feel like my whole life is turned inside out and nothing makes sense anymore. I don't know what is important anymore. I've turned into this dead thing that is alive [...]; my apartment feels like the inside of a coffin. I can't tell anybody I have this, I can't tell anybody anything. I imagine them looking at me funny. I see them pulling away from me, from my body; I feel poisoned. My body is poisoned. I feel diseased, I feel like something that needs to be taken out into the desert and shot. But I'm too scared to do the shooting. At first I wanted to die but now I just want to live. I want to be left alone so I can live my life in peace, but how can I be alone with this thing ... how can I be alone with this?" (126)

Sheila, the facilitator of the group consoles Rayna: '"No, Rayna, none of us has to go through this alone. That's why we're here" (127). Sherman suggests that support group serves as a substitute for 'family' for HIV- positive people.

Rayna then tells her adoptive parents Circe and Car and her friend C'Anne about her HIV infection. The love and care of her parents and friends boost up her courage for sometime. However, she develops a "growing anger [...] toward HIV-negative people" (164). Finally, she speaks to Theodore who accepts her infection easily. In course of their conversation, he reveals that he always gets himself tested for AIDS every year, is negative so far and that his own brother Powell being deliberately shunned by his family because of his gayness had died from AIDS all alone. Even Theodore himself called his brother '"a punk'" (169). He has been living with a terrible sense of guilt, since he '"didn't do nothing, didn't say nothing, didn't visit, didn't call, nothing"' (169). Homosexual AIDS that was once looked upon with bigotry is juxtaposed with heterosexual AIDS that is seen with tolerance just because it affects the hegemonic community. Theodore then forces reluctant Rayna to meet Mrs. Jenkins, whose husband developed AIDS following his occasional drug use and his unsafe sexual practices with multiple partners, and subsequently died from the disease. To memorialize her husband with whom she had spent twenty-five years as wife, Mrs. Jenkins, with the insurance money she received after his death started her Dancing Unicorn House, a kind of home for the children with AIDS. Theodore regularly visits Jenkins and spends his time with kids to overcome his guilt. He therefore insists that Rayna should go there to lessen the burden of her fear and grief. Nevertheless, Rayna's logic is "How do you look into the eyes of a dying child and stay sane?"(172). Eventually Theodore's caressing touch changes Rayna's attitude to HIV-positive life, as she confesses in her journal:

> We don't have to be afraid of loving, he said.

> This is not the time to be without touch, he said. Now is when we need it more than ever. And I'm not talking about sex, I'm talking about touch, he said.
>
> He took my hands in his and kissed them. [...] He trailed his tongue along the inside of my thigh and I started to squirm.
>
> You want me to stop? He asked.
>
> [...]
>
> [...]. Don't stop, I said, [...]. I am alive and a sensual being. I am entitled to this pleasure.
>
> I felt so alive beneath the warmth of his breath. His lips made me think about anything but death.
>
> [...]
>
> [...] I was astride him and able to ride until I reached a land where there was no AIDS, no terror, no secrets, only this grinding pleasure, this wicked wetness between my legs.
>
> And that's just a taste of what safer sex can be like, he said.
>
> We lay on that rug for hours breathing together, licking, rubbing, holding, being still. It was as if the HIV had broken something open in our relationship; there was no room for lying or secrets. There was not even space for promises. Those, I told him, are forbidden. He made me promise to meet Mrs. Jenkins and her kids, though. So I will do it. For myself and for Theodore.
>
> How could I say no to a man who can caress me with words like that? (172-74)

Sherman highlights the fact that heterosexual HIV-positive life can be full of love and pleasure. She also rejects the abstinence theory of the rightist in the sexual epidemic. As the days pass, Rayna's sex life with Theodore takes an exciting, invigorating turn:

> Now, Theodore sleeps with me most nights and wraps me inside his arms [...] as I dream of death.
>
> [...]
>
> Theodore touches me. [...] we are still able to be intimate. How I've grown to love surgical gloves and have found a certain kind of sexiness in latex. A little lube inside a rubber can go a long way. [...] dental dams do feel like silk stockings.
>
> All it takes is an imagination. And Theodore has plenty of that. (201)

Safety in HIV/AIDS does not mean denial of bodily pleasure and intimacy. It is rather a necessary virtue that seeks to fortify life and love against the threat of AIDS. Theodore becomes a turning point in Rayna's HIV-positive life. Rayna's focus is now shifted to the activist group as she realizes the justness of its protest. She starts collecting evidence against Dr. Van Horne who, ever since the Latosha Briggs case, had been sterilizing poor HIV-positive women without their consent and yet was backed by the hospital. She plans to copy from the confidential doctors' files the consent forms bearing false signatures of the sterilized patients and to pass them over to the activist group Prejudice Posse that is fighting for the Briggs's case. Though she knows that her doing would amount to a crime, she takes a decision to go ahead with her plan. Her conscience pricks her: "Innocent women were having their privacy invaded, their rights taken away. All because of the virus in their blood. The same virus that ran wild through her blood" (177). A fighter's spirit possesses her. Contrastingly, Rayna herself does not want to experience pregnancy and motherhood, considering her own HIV-positive status. This is evident when she responds to C'Anne who suggests:

> " Maybe you and Theodore will have a baby,"[...].
>
> "I couldn't do that to the child or to myself. If the child is negative then I risk leaving it motherless, and if it's positive I could never forgive myself. And I know Theodore wouldn't go along with it. He could get infected by having unprotected sex with me. And then we'd all have the peculiar pleasure of watching each other die. I couldn't even stand the thought."(184)

Through an HIV-positive black woman, Sherman wants to rationalize HIV-positive Black women's desire for motherhood. Despite her sharp rational insight, Rayna sees Dr. Horne's practice of deterring someone by force from enjoying the right to motherhood as an unjust act. She therefore decides to expose the doctor. With Novel's help, she locates at their hospital two sterilized HIV-positive women's files, gets them copied and mails them to the Prejudice Posse. On top of it, obeying Theodore's advice, she visits Mrs. Jenkins's Dancing Unicorn House and intends to spend time painting with HIV-positive kids there: "'I'm going to find a way to show them how art can help them to understand life'" (183). Even as she does all these things, she feels the need of the honest people's company around her to be spiritually resurrected:

> [...]. I need people in my life who are going to tell me the truth. I don't have any time left for lies.
>
> I've been stripped down to my bones. [...] I could be called leper, whore, junkie, bloodsucker, dyke, Rayna, unholy one. None of those names matters. I have been stripped. I have been cleansed. In the icy grip of death, I have been reborn. (187)

In her acceptance of the inevitable, Rayna demonstrates

her stoic endurance of and calm attitude towards her own HIV-positive life. She wants to live meaningfully now. Despite sore throat, she conducts her art workshop among the HIV- positive children at Mrs. Jenkins's where she meets a girl named Anika who has full-blown AIDS. She draws the picture of a person representing an ancestor, and teaches the children a lesson on immortality:

> "[...]. In some places in the world, people believe that we are not brand-new when we're born, but that we are our ancestors, reborn. That the thoughts and lives of our ancestors are woven inside us and in that way our ancestors live on inside us. That way there is no death and no one ever really dies."
>
> "Like my mama isn't really dead?" Anika asked.
>
> "Not as long as you remember her, she's not. She'll always live on inside you."
>
> "And when we die someone will remember us?" Enuya asked.
>
> "Yes, and then you'll always live on inside them. And it goes on and on like that forever."(191)

Rayna's attempt to instil in the dying children a sense of eternal life is indicative of her spirit to defy at least mental, if not physical death from AIDS. By spending lot of time with the children, Rayna gradually develops her sense of well-being and feels specially attached to Anika: "[...] Anika [...] is in the late stages of the disease. [...] She clings to me like a second skin while I'm there" (192). Anika wants Rayna to be her mother. However, Rayna is not prepared for that, as "she was afraid of mothers" (195). As a child, she was left uncared-for by her own mother who was a mental patient. Moreover, she herself has lost her motherhood due to the several abortions she has had since she was nineteen years of age. However, the thought of her adoptive parents Car and Circe who had loved her enough changes her mind, "Whatever it takes to mother this child, I'll do" (199). She has also other intention: "[...] she would not be one of the people in Anika's life who would lie to her. [...] She would help her face the truth of her situation, unflinchingly" (198). At last, she decides to adopt Anika, to give the latter a home full of love. However, her plan does not materialize as Anika dies within weeks. Through Anika, Sherman brings out the poignant picture of children with AIDS and in doing so discourages HIV- positive women's desire for motherhood.

After Anika's death, Rayna breaks down completely. Following the incident, grief-stricken Rayna's spirit to fight the illegal and brutal practices of the hospital administration revives. With Novel's assistance, she finds the Van Horne files, from which she collects more information. She decides to send the details to the Prejudice Posse to help them in their fight against the doctor's discrimination. She wants to undo the unchallengeable hegemony of Van Horne who "was still walking around the place like he owned it and God" (206). Now she is not even afraid of losing her job, "What do I have to lose that hasn't already been lost?"(206).

In the last chapter of the book, C'Anne, Novel and Rayna hug each other in a park as they laugh loudly over the suggestion to be together always. Theodore figures only in their conversation as their '"homeboy"' (213) who still loves Rayna. Their laughter is "Loud and deep enough for Anika to hear" (214). Anika is internalized in Rayna so much so that the former becomes an objectification of the latter's condition. Anika was innocent, had AIDS and died from the disease. Rayna is equally innocent, has AIDS and will die from the disease. Perhaps Sherman wants her readers to see this. She draws a parallel between them through loud and deep laughter. In other words, Sherman suggests that Anika represents the stereotypical notion of 'innocent victim' of AIDS. Laughter undoes this cultural construction and thereby projects Rayna as the innocent one. In fact, all are innocent in so far as AIDS infection is concerned. The novelist therefore wants the HIV-positive people to laugh their disease off, to refuse to accept themselves as stigmatists. Hence it is logical on her part to end her novel with Rayna writing in her diary that "those who love me will be there, holding my hand, urging me forward and loving me, as I step from the light of this world into the darkness of the next" (214).

Loving touch has the force and power to energize Rayna who in turn develops a positive attitude towards her life, and recognizes her HIV-positive identity as something dignified and meaningful. Sherman totally breaks the hegemonic binary thinking in relation to HIV/AIDS.

The above four HIV/AIDS novels seek to depict the affirmation of HIV positive identity through resistance to the hegemonic and dominant notions of the disease.

5

Conclusion

With the slowdown of mortality from HIV/AIDS at the moment, this chapter seeks to revisit briefly the cultural perceptions and interpretations concerning the disease that have been examined in the preceding chapters. In so doing, it also proposes to highlight what might be called "the sites of non-prevention theory" of the disease in the preceding three decades.

The notion of categorization in our society entails inclusion of some people by exclusion of others. Exclusion then is justified through "stigma" that aims at disgracing either the categorized or the non-categorized. Categorization is always projected as a "natural" thing whereas, in actuality, it is socially constructed. We, the people love to categorize ourselves perhaps just to privilege "us" over "them" or "the other." We love to construct such binaries just to hierarchize ourselves. We love to be at the centre by constructing the peripheries. In order to be dominant and hegemonic, we love to create around ourselves myths or images or superlatives that are intended for public consumption. In our relentless pursuit of our images, we have lost our own selves. Our tendency to label something or somebody comes out of our ideologies and prejudices that are often normative or regulatory rather than rational or non-judgemental.

Unprejudiced HIV/AIDS discourse challenges the very notion of categorization or binarization and of what might be called "normative society" by exploring the brutal truth (be it essential or social), by intruding into the closest distance between human bodies and into the innermost human affairs. From the vantage point of normative society, the human body is looked at as something that must be healthy, beautiful, male, erotic (whereas the female body must be procreative, since motherhood is compulsory), heterosexual, monogamous (even though scriptural Gods, prophets and characters who are worshipped in some religions are having many licit or illicit sexual partners) and familial. Failure to conform to these norms attracts vituperation leading to ostracization, excommunication and stigmatization of the human body. Unbiased HIV/AIDS discourse has been able to counter these norms both clinically and non-clinically by bringing to the surface the cultural politics embedded in them. It has also raised certain epistemological questions concerning HIV positive identity that, in effect, have helped change the popular perception of the disease and the diseased. Consequently, the epidemic spread of the disease has been curbed.

Sociology of HIV/AIDS has often engaged itself more with the interpretative community of the disease than with the HIV positive people, and thereby engendered linguistic and social construction theories that have eventually resulted, to a certain extent, in the non-prevention of the epidemic. In the "representation" of HIV/AIDS, it has always sought affiliations with ideologies that privilege the normative and regulatory over the rational and non-judgmental. In the past years, it had mostly used metaphoric and metonymic languages that had sociopolitical implications. For example, "tsunami," "time bomb," "holocaust," "apocalypse," "invasion," "collective calamity," and "plague" were very frequently used for the HIV/AIDS epidemic. "Victim," "enemy," "the other," "alien," "pariah," and "outcast" had been much in vogue for the HIV positive person whose condition had always been referred to as something that was "stigmatizing." "War" was used for prevention and control. These terms, as Susan Sontag in her book *AIDS and Its Metaphors* suggests, with their predominantly martial connotation had projected the disease as something that was devastating (45-94). Coupled with these tropes was the notion of 'stigma.' Stigma is something that historically inheres in all sexually transmitted diseases including HIV/AIDS. All these in turn caused panic that was made interchangeable with plague in dominant discourse in its urgent need for the dramatic search for the magic bullets for the epidemic. This gave ubiquitous status to the disease and inspired fears of easy transmission through even non-transmissible routes such as transmission through sharing drinking cups, glasses, pens, toothbrushes, towels, beds, public toilet seats and so on.

HIV/AIDS was perceived to deserve "serious" attention only when it affected the famous people, the posh localities, and the rich or powerful nations. "AIDS" would never have become a household word in the West, had there been no death of Rock Hudson, a Hollywood movie star from the disease in 1985 in America. Validation of the existence of disease including HIV/AIDS through the rich, the powerful, and the well-known is culturally written in the public unconscious. Corollarily, a celebrity was mostly chosen in the mass media as the agent of publicizing and popularizing the HIV/AIDS prevention so as to goad the people into awareness. This was understood as deep 'concern' even as the callousness of the society was palpably felt by the HIV-positive people then.

Frequent inept engagement with the foreign origin theories that attempted to locate the origin of HIV/AIDS elsewhere and in the others like gays, Africans, prostitutes, city-dwellers, and non-natives as against heterosexuals, non-Africans, wives, country people, and natives served only to divert attention from the prevention to the proliferation of the disease. It always sought to hierarchize and dichotomize the incidence and distribution of the disease. This happened in the last two decades of the 20th century.

Most of the help organizations (for example, NGOs) that were mushrooming initially in the name of the HIV/ AIDS prevention and awareness often proclaimed dedicated service to HIV positive people with the sole intention to be in the limelight. In so doing, they attracted huge resources from international or national sources that were generating enormous funds to be utilized for the dissemination of knowledge about the prevention of the disease. The organizational members often embezzled the donated moneys.

Pharmacists often violated their ethics or promises of preserving secrecy of the identities of HIV-positive customers who were blackmailed or compelled to buy medicines at prices unreasonably higher than the actual costs. Their moneymaking theory dissuaded many poor HIV positive people who failed to enter into bargain from taking medicines. Most of the doctors then had either refused to visit AIDS patients who were acutely ill or frequently charged higher fees for each visit. Some doctors justified the transmission of the disease to themselves in the process of their involvement with treatment of the ill and the scarcity of such resources as their time and hospital beds for the sick. These justifications were coupled with the suggestion that undergoing treatment was wastage of time and money on the part of the infected on grounds of the absolute certainty of their death from HIV/AIDS. Some physicians, as a result of negotiations with political leaders and public health authorities that considered issues like "incentives" offered to treat HIV positive patients and to take risks, entered into a "contract." The contract protected their interests such as salary advance, reimbursement for travelling and living expenses, promise of promotion, transfer to a place of doctor's choice, access to research funds in addition to huge cash rewards and so on. They made money, status and opportunities legally or illegally out of the HIV/AIDS epidemic.

As always, 'abstinence,' 'monogamy' and 'family' are also prescribed as prevention formulas to date. However, abstinence that is often preached as a prevention strategy is seen to be the theory of the diehard moral majority, is considered impractical and is mostly honoured in indulgence. Monogamy as a prophylactic apparatus is viewed as the irrational theory of the rabid right. Monogamy is, as the left would argue, often respected either in the breach or in adultery in the absence of easy serial monogamy or of polygamy or polyandry. Family as a preventive is reckoned as something that is erotically unconvincing. Family, as the feminists and gay theorists argue, meets only the procreative needs without having any notion of desire and pleasure and hence promotes the interest of patriarchy. It defines manhood and womanhood in terms of the ability for impregnation and pregnancy. For the live-in partners (of both the same and opposite sexes), marital or family life is bondage. For the mobile and multiple sex partners, family makes no sense, is just a social label that rather serves to hide promiscuity.

According to heterosexual, patriarchal and pro-family perceptions, anonymous sex with woman is possible "only" either by force or on payment. However, forcible sexual intercourse otherwise termed as rape that also rules out the role of HIV preventives is not always possible on juridical and social grounds. This is the reason why, as the feminists allege, the term "prostitutes" (though it is now replaced by the polite and non-discriminatory phrase "commercial sex workers") is historically and judgmentally constructed with the intention to project women as a category that sells their bodies to men. The term is also politically intended to keep intact the respectability of words such as wife, mother, sister and daughter. On top of all, culturally women who were ironically exempted from being the carriers of HIV/AIDS in the 1980s in America following the gayness of the illness have always been regarded as the diseased in the history of diseases. The prostitutes rather than unsafe sex practices are shown as the source of infection. Man's infection with HIV is always shown as having its origin in woman. If the husband transmits the disease to his wife, then the former all on a sudden is exculpated and the latter is inculpated and interpreted as a promiscuous, corrupt woman. Culturally, all venereal diseases target woman for stigmatization that ranges from, among other things, the threat of assaults by the distraught family members and neighbours to homicide.

Prophylactic theory demands sex with the mediation of technology. It entails "conscious" preparation for the use of technology whose presence in the genital area also continues to linger in awareness right at the time of coition. This is seen as barrier between bodies, desires and orgasmic pleasures. This is understood as threat to masculinity and femininity in heterosexual matrix that perceives, as the AIDS cultural critic Tamsin Wilton in her book *Engendering AIDS* argues, the ability to have unmediated "penis-in-vagina ejaculation" as "real, adult sex"(34). Hence, there is disinclination for condom use. Moreover, the feminists view male condom as a phallocentric thing. The female condom is seen as the empowerment of women by men. Its use, as the argument goes, fully protects women against infection with STDs and HIV/AIDS, despite any unsafe or irresponsible sex with them by men who for their harmful practices have to be concerned about their exposure to risk. This safety guard for women is not well tolerated by men. Particularly women whose only source of livelihood is to have sex with their customers on payment are often threatened with violence and abandonment by men. These ideological interpretations seek to discourage condom use. Non-penetrative sex is understood as foreplay. There is aversion to the use of dental dam by lesbians, since they are not yet convinced that HIV/AIDS can affect them. Throwing away a needle after its single use to keep HIV from being transmitted through the blood is often felt as breach of intimacy and as monotonous practice by IV-drug users who usually enjoy sharing only one needle in their circles of friends, cannot wait for anything to sate their insatiable urge for addiction. On top of all, education on the use of prophylactics in public is seen as condonation of indiscriminate and illegal sexual practices, drug use in different age groups. With the recent rise in sexual practices among children under 15 years of age, sex education in public might be discouraged.

These cultural determinants of HIV/AIDS have begot non-prevention theory and, in the process, prevented the HIV-positive people from being understood appropriately with love and care. The above discussion in the light of the study made in the preceding chapters of this book, by and large, seeks to give the picture of the hegemonic notion and the politics of the disease then and now.

The study therefore shows, first of all, that disease, be it experienced or perceived, is always a linguistic (metaphoric and metonymic) product, since the entire world, after all, is understood through language. Richard Gwyn puts it succinctly:

> Illness is constructed, reproduced and perpetuated through language. We get to know about our own illnesses through the language of doctors and nurses, friends and relatives, and we often recycle the words picked up from our consultations in the doctor's surgery into conversation, sprinkling our stories of sickness with epithets that give the impression of a grander knowledge of medical science. When we open the newspapers or switch on the television or radio, we encounter an increasing variety of articles and programmes offering information, advice and warnings about

> every conceivable dimension of health and care of the body. (6)

When this linguistic presentation of disease in the form of events that take place within and across time is purposefully made in "sequence" or "order," disease narrative comes into being.

As with all types of narratives, disease narratives then involve stories. As has been discussed in Chapter-I, the telling and hearing of stories are very crucial to the understanding and framing of human experiences. Stories serve as indispensable testimony to validate individual identities. At this point, it would be appropriate to quote A. Kerby who rightly points out, "The stories we tell are part and parcel of our becoming. They are a mode of vision, plotting what is good and what is bad for us, what is possible and what is not - plotting who we may become. But in the telling we seem also to be immediately involved in generating the *value* of a certain state of affairs or course of action, of judging its worth, ethical or otherwise" (53). Thus, stories by and large, seek affiliations with ideologies that are at once normative or regulatory and rational or non-judgmental. It has also been the case with disease narratives in which the experiences of the pathologized bodies, minds and social lives of human beings under the impact of terminal or chronic diseases are framed and understood through illness stories. In other words, illness finds voice through narrativisation of it in disease narratives. As Kleinman points out, "The illness narrative is a story the patient tells, and significant others retell, to give coherence to the distinctive events and long term course of suffering. The plot lines, core metaphors, and rhetorical devices that structure the illness narrative are drawn from cultural and personal models for arranging experiences in meaningful ways and for effectively communicating those meanings. Over the long course of chronic disorder, these model texts shape and even create experience. The personal narrative does not merely reflect illness experience, but rather it contributes to the experience of symptoms and suffering" (49).

There has been a spurt of "illness narratives" in the West especially following HIV/AIDS since the late 1980s. This kind of fascination with writing HIV/AIDS stories (nonfictional and fictional) can be attributable to the complexity and fatality of the disease and to the Western obsession with the theme of reflexiveness, disclosure and discovery of the self and identity. In the preceding chapters (II, III and IV), American HIV/AIDS nonfictional and fictional narratives have been examined to demonstrate that HIV/AIDS discourse is an open-ended thing or subject which fails to answer appropriately the crucial question of HIV-positive identity that is a conflation of endless chaos and quest. The chaos happens as a result of surrendering to hegemonic notion. It brings about negation of selfhood, whereas the quest energetically engages itself with challenging the dominant notion, thereby causing affirmation of identity. This process of conflict between continuity and change in human perception about HIV/AIDS will linger as long as the cure is not available. However, the book has the ethical intention of providing insights into the meanings and experiences of the disease. This insight might benefit patients, healthcare provider, doctors and, of course, people who might hypothesize again with new perspectives by challenging the existing notion. HIV/AIDS is a disease that requires both clinical and nonclinical interventions to curb its spread. This book aims at intervening nonmedically and intellectually as well in the popular perception of the disease as stigma.

Bibliography

Albert, Edward. "The Response of the Press to AIDS." *The Social Dimensions of AIDS: Method and Theory.* Ed.
Douglas A. Feldman and Thomas M. Johnson. New York: Praeger, 1986. 163-78.

Althusser, Louis. "Ideology and Ideological State Apparatuses (Notes towards an Investigation)." *Mapping Ideology.* Ed. Slavoj Zizek. London: Verso, 1994. 100-40.

Atkinson, Karen, and Rob Midlehurst. "Representing AIDS: the textual politics of health discourse." *Theorizing Culture: An Interdisciplinary Critique After Postmodernism.* Ed. Barbara Adam and Stuart Allan. New York: New York University Press, 1995. 113-28.

Benveniste, Emile. *Problems in General Linguistcs.* Trans. Mary Elizabeth Meek. Coral Gables: University of Miami Press, 1971.

Bersani, Leo. "Is the Rectum a Grave?" *October* 43 (1987): 197-222.

Bleuler, Manfred. "What is Schizophrenia?" *Schizophrenia Bulletin* 10 (1984):8.

Bourjaily, Vance. *Old Soldier.* New York: Donald I. Fine, Inc., 1990.

Brandt, Allan M. "AIDS: From Social History to Social Policy." *AIDS: The Burdens of History.* Ed. Elizabeth Fee and Daniel M. Fox. Berkeley: University of California Press, 1988. 147-71.

Brodkey, Harold. *This Wild Darkness: The Story of My Death.* New York:Metropolitan, 1996.

Brooks, Peter. *Reading for the Plot: Design and Intention in Narrative.* Oxford: Clarendon Press, 1984.

Buchanan, Ian. *A Dictionary of Critical Theory.* New York: Oxford University Press, 2010.

Butler, Judith. *Bodies that Matter: On the Discursive Limits of "Sex."* New York: Routledge, 1993.

Butler, Judith. *Gender Trouble: Feminism and the Subversion of Identity.* New York: Routledge, 1990.

Collins, Patricia Hill. *Black Sexual Politics: African Americans,Gender, and the New Racism.* New York: Routledge,
2004.

Crimp, Douglas. "AIDS: Cultural Analysis/Cultural Activism." *October* 43 (1987): 3-16.

Crimp, Douglas. "How to Have Promiscuity in an Epidemic." *October* 43 (1987): 237-71.

Culler, Jonathan. *On Deconstruction: Theory and Criticism after Structuralism.* Ithaca: Cornell University Press, 1982.

Davis, Christopher. *Philadelphia.* New York: Bantam, 1993.

Derrida, Jacques. *Of Grammatology.* Trans. Gayatri Chakravorty Spivak. Baltimore: Johns Hopkins University Press, 1976.

Donne, John. *Devotions Upon Emergent Occasions.*1623. Rpt. in *The Complete Poetry and Selected Prose of John Donne.* Ed. Charles M. Coffin. New York: Modern Library, 1952.

Douglas, Mary. *Risk and Blame.* London: Routledge, 1992.

Durant, Penny Raife. *When Heroes Die.* New York: Aladdin, 1992.

Edgar, Andrew. "body." *Key Concepts in Cultural Theory.* Ed. Andrew Edgar and Peter Sedgwick. London: Routledge, 2004. 44-47.

Foucault, Michel. *Discipline and Punish: The Birth of the Prison.* Trans. Alan Sheridan. Harmondsworth: Penguin, 1979.

Foucault, Michel. *The History of Sexuality: Volume 1 An Introduction.* Trans. Robert Hurley. London: Penguin, 1981.

Fumento, Michael. Rev. of *And the Band Played On,* by Randy Shilts. *American Spectator* Feb. 1988. 24 August 2005 url:<http://www.Michael Fumento reviews And the Band Played On. htm>

Fuss, Diana. *Essentially Speaking: Feminism, Nature & Difference.* New York: Routledge, 1989.

Gilman, Sander L. *Disease and Representation.* Ithaca: Cornell University Press, 1988.

Garmire, Lisa. "Resisting the Apocalypse: Telling Time in American Novels about AIDS, 1982-1992." Doctoral Diss. UCSB, 1996. 23 November 2005 <http://E:\rips projects\novels\Paul Monette's AIDS Novels-Lisa Garmire, UCSB Dissertation,1996.htm>

Grover, Jan Zita. "AIDS: Keywords." *October* 43 (1987): 17-30.

Gwyn, Richard. *Communicating Health and Illness.* London: Sage, 2002.

"HIV Cases on the Rise among Youth." *Times of India* 3 June. 2008: 6.

Hoffman, Alice. *At Risk.* New York: Putnam, 1988.

Hogan, Katie. "Speculations on Women and AIDS." *Minnesota Review* 40 (1993): 84-93.

Kerby, A. *Narrative and the Self.* Bloomington: Indiana University Press, 1991.

Kerr, M.E. *Night Kites.* Cambridge: Harper and Row Publishers, 1986.

Kleinman, A. *The Illness Narratives.* New York: Basic Books, 1988.

Kruger, Steven F. *AIDS Narratives: Gender and Sexuality, Fiction and Science.* New York: Garland, 1996.

Laclau, Ernesto, ed. *The Making of Political Identities.* New York: Verso, 1994.

Laplanche J., and J.B. Pontalis. *The Language of Psycho-Analysis.* London: Hogarth Press, 1983.

Marcus, Laura. *Auto/biographical Discourses: Theory, Criticism, Practice.* Manchester: Manchester University Press, 1994.

Meltzer, Francoise. "Unconscious." *Critical Terms for Literary Study.* Ed. Frank Lentricchia and Thomas McLaughlin. Chicago: The University of Chicago Press, 1990. 147-62.

Miklowitz, Gloria D. *Good-bye Tomorrow.* New York: Laurel-Leaf Books, 1987.

Milner, Andrew, and Jeff Browitt., Ed. *Contemporary Cultural Theory: An Introduction.* 3rd ed. London: Routledge, 2002.

Mitchell, W. J. T. *Iconology: Image, Text, Ideology.* Chicago: The Chicago University Press, 1986.

Mitchell, W. J. T. "Representation." *Critical Terms for Literary Study.* Ed. Frank Lentricchia and Thomas McLaughlin. Chicago: The University of Chicago Press, 1990. 11-22.

Monette, Paul. *Borrowed Time: An AIDS Memoir.* New York: Avon Books, 1988.

Monette, Paul. *Afterlife.* New oYork: Crown Publishers, Inc., 1990.

Moya, Paula M. L. Introduction. *Reclaiming Identity: Realist Theory and the Predicament of Postmodernism.* Ed. Paula M. L. Moya and Michael R. Hames-Garcia. Hyderabad: Orient Longman, 2001. 1-26.

Moya, Paula M.L. "Postmodernism, 'Realism,' and the Politics of Identity: Cherrie Moraga and Chicana Feminism." *Reclaiming Identity: Realist Theory and the*

Predicament of Postmodernism. Ed. Paula M. L. Moya and Michael R. Hames-Garcia. Hyderabad: Orient Longman, 2001. 67-101.

Nietzsche, Friedrich. *On the Genealogy of Morals.* Trans. Walter Kaufmann. New York: Vintage, 1969.

Patton, Cindy. *Globalizing AIDS.* Minneapolis: University of Minnesota Press, 2002.

Patton, Cindy. *Inventing AIDS.* New York: Routledge, 1990.

Peirce, Charles Sanders. *Collected Papers.* eds. Charles Hartshorne and Paul Weiss. 8 vols. Cambridge: Harvard University Press, 1931.

Ricoeur, Paul. *Oneself as Another.* Trans. Kathleen Blamey. Chicago: The University of Chicago Press, 1992.

Sarup, Madan. *Identity, Culture and the Postmodern World.* Ed. Tasneem Raja. 1996. Edinburgh: Edinburgh University Press, 2002.

Sedgwick, Eve Kosofsky. *Between Men: English Literature and Male Homosocial Desire.* New York: Columbia University Press, 1985.

Sheldon, Sally. "The Masculine Body." *Real Bodies: A Sociological Introduction.* Ed. Mary Evans and Ellie Lee. New York: Palgrave, 2002. 14-28.

Sherman, Charlotte Watson. *Touch.* New York: Harper Perennial, 1995.

Shilts, Randy. *And the Band Played On: Politics, People, and the AIDS Epidemic.* New York: Penguin, 1988.

Silverman, Kaja. *The Subject of Semiotics.* New York: Oxford University Press, 1983.

Singer, Linda. *Erotic Welfare: Sexual Theory and Politics in the Age of Epidemic.* Ed. Judith Butler and Maureen MacGrogan. New York: Routledge, 1993.

Sontag, Susan. *AIDS and Its Metaphors.* New York: Farrar, 1989.

Stroll, Avrum. "Identity." *Encyclopaedia of Philosophy.* ed. Paul Edwards. Vol . 4. New York: Macmillan/Free press, 1967.

Thomas, Carol. "The 'Disabled' Body." *Real Bodies: A Sociological Introduction.* Ed. Mary Evans and Ellie Lee. New York: Palgrave, 2002. 64-78.

Treichler, Paula A. *How to Have Theory in an Epidemic.* Durham: Duke University Press, 1999.

Verghese, Abraham. *My Own Country: A Doctor's Story.* New Delhi: Penguin Books, 1998.

"Viral Tsunami: Unchecked HIV epidemic could destroy countries." Editorial. *Times of India* 8 Jan. 2005: 8.

Watney, Simon. *Policing Desire: Pornography, AIDS, and the Media.* Minneapolis: University of Minnesota Press, 1987.

Watney, Simon. *Practices of Freedom: Selected Writings on HIV/AIDS.* Durham: Duke University Press, 1994.

Wendell, S. *The Rejected Body: Feminist Philosophical Reflections on Disability.* London: Routledge, 1996.

Williams, Raymond. *Keywords: A Vocabulary of Culture and Society.* Rev. ed. New York: Oxford University Press, 1983.

Williams, S., and G. Bendelow. *The Lived Body: Sociological Themes, Embodied Issues.* London: Routledge, 1998.

Wilton, Tamsin. *EnGendering AIDS.* London: Sage, 1997.

Wittgenstein, Ludwig. *Culture and Value.* Trans. Peter Winch. Oxford: Basil Blackwell, 1980.

Woodward, Kath, Ed. *Questioning Identity: Gender, Class, Ethnicity.* London: Routledge, 2004.

World Health Organization. *Understanding and Living with AIDS.* New Delhi: World Health Organization Regional Office for South-East Asia, 1992.

Yingling, Thomas E. *AIDS and the National Body.* Ed. Robyn Wiegman. Durham: Duke University Press, 1997.

Index